Words of V
for yo
Health & Happiness!

101 ARTICLES, QUESTIONS & ANSWERS
ON NATURAL HEALTH

BY BREDA GARDNER

www.bredagardner.com

Edited, compiled & title by Jerry Gardner

Words of Wisdom for your Health & Happiness written by Breda Gardner

Photos by Karen Cunningham, reproduced by kind permission.
www.karencphotography.ie

Cover and Canine Photos by Jerry Gardner
Cover Photo: Sunrise over Waimanalo Beach, Hawaii

Publication designed & printed by Applied Image.
www.appliedimage.ie

Published by Applied Image.

ACKNOWLEDGEMENT

I dedicate this book to my husband and soul-mate Jerry. Thanks to his constant support, encouragement and belief in me, this book flowed easily and effortlessly. I thank him from the bottom of my heart for making my life purpose an easy journey.

I would like to thank the many practitioners, teachers, family members, friends and clients too numerous to mention who have encouraged and helped me over the years. Special thanks to Jan de Vries for his kind foreword and to Karen Cunningham for her beautiful photos.

I would also like to thank the following: my four children, Físonn, Orla, Ciara and Iona for their ongoing love and laughter. John Andrews for his continuous support and for his unconditional sharing of his passion and knowledge in iridology. Roger Dyson for his in-depth knowledge of homeopathy and diagnostic kinesiology, and for his generosity in giving me clinical experience in his London practice. Dr. Patricia O'Toole for helping to restore my faith in GP's. Colin Turner of Applied Image for his inspired design of this book.

Throughout the book I have used a selection of my favourite quotations. I have not always been able to remember where they are from, so my apologies – and thanks! – to the people who have provided these wonderful words. Here are two lines which reflect my view on life, and which underscore my belief that a positive outlook is central to our health and well-being:

"Live well, laugh often and love much." Bessie Anderson Stanley

"When you think everything is someone else's fault, you will suffer a lot. When you realize that everything springs only from yourself, you will learn both peace and joy." The Dalai Lama

Breda.

FOREWORD BY JAN DE VRIES

It was a great privilege to be asked to do a foreword for this book. Personally I feel that this is a book that should be in every household! The writer has used her knowledge and her gifts to provide clear and concise information to the reader to help them lead a healthier life.

We live in a very busy society, which has brought its problems, and due to economic growth it has put extra burdens on people's lives. With methods written in this book it is evident that releasing these burdens can be done. We are grateful for experienced practitioners who, in this very busy world, understand the task of how to meet people's needs.

I have followed Breda's career and know that she is a great practitioner using disciplines that give her the ability to find the right diagnosis and the right remedies to help each individual's needs.

This book is yet another step to building bridges between orthodox and alternative medicine, which is leading towards Complementary Medicine. There is a great need for this today and both fields of medicine should be working together to find the best system to help human suffering.

Personally I have been 50 years in practice and I am happy to have seen this growth. Academic practitioners are just as much in need of practical practitioners and my experience has shown how well it can work together. We cannot afford to lose the wisdom in treating patients. Breda's book fills a gap in the practicalities that are necessary to treat illness and disease.

My friend Hans Moolenburgh said that having been an orthodox GP, he found the medical practice harsh and got a feeling that they know it all. He often said that orthodox was Yang (male) and alternative medicine was Ying (female), which was more friendly, gentle and probably with a little bit extra care. As he always said, it is time Ying and Yang get together. Luckily in this day and age that is happening and we see so much evidence in this book of that. That is why this book is so special and encouraging.

Prof. Jan de Vries ND, MRN, DAc, MBAcA, DSc.
Auchenkyle Clinic
Southwood Road
Troon
Scotland

INTRODUCTION

When I started writing a natural health column for the Waterford Today newspaper in back in March 2005, little did I imagine I would be here some three years later publishing a compilation of 101 of the best received articles. This book has come about as a result of synchronicity in my life's journey, and the articles are based on:

- **My experiences with clients in my complementary health clinics in Kilkenny and Waterford (my clients ask questions on a daily basis!).**
- **Questions and feedback from readers of my columns in the Carlow First, Kilkenny Advertiser and Waterford Today newspapers.**
- **Feedback from the regular positive living workshops and homeopathic first aid courses I organise.**
- **15 years spent working as a nurse in Ireland, the UK, the USA and the Middle East.**
- **Working and talking with my fellow health practitioners and teachers.**
- **My own intuition guiding me on how to help people to be more comfortable with themselves and with others.**

My background is in nursing: I worked as a nurse for 15 years, and loved it. However, when I was in my early twenties, I suffered from endogenous depression for three years. I became incapacitated towards work and towards the outside world. Nothing prepared me for the downward spiral of gloom and sadness I felt inside my body. I was so unaware as to why I was feeling this way. My psychiatrist had put me on anti-depressants. These had shifted my chemical imbalance, but I was suffering terrible side effects - like high blood pressure, skin allergies, headaches and constipation - and I still felt numb inside me.

In the midst of this suppressed state brought on by the anti-depressants, I cried out for help – but each time I attended my GP, he would just reassure me that I looked great and so should be feeling better. I felt extremely disillusioned and that my voice was not being heard. Just because I looked fine on the outside didn't mean I wasn't feeling pain inside my body. Then one day whilst in Dublin, I found myself being guided to visit Eason's book centre. I found a book called "Your Erroneous Zones" by Dr Wayne Dyer. This book was my saviour (for more, see the article entitled "The Book That Changed My Life"). Finally I felt there was someone out there who really understood – and who really felt – what I was going through.

Reading the book made me more aware of myself, my feelings and my emotions – but most importantly, it gave me guidance on how to move on. I came off my medication and began to put into practice what the book advised: I kept a gratitude journal, and wrote down positive affirmations on a daily basis. The advice in the book helped me to change my negative thoughts into more positive ones. And as my mental energy improved, I noticed that my physical energy became better day by day. Conventional medicine alone had not worked for me: I needed something more.

On my 24th birthday, I therefore made a vow to myself that I would learn as much as I could about health and well-being so that I would never again have to experience this dark side of living. I moved to London and spent 15 years there, ten of them studying a range of natural and complementary therapies, including exercise to music, massage therapy, aromatherapy, kinesiology (muscle-testing), iridology and finally homeopathy. Because of what I had been through, I felt I had found new ways of applying all of these therapies to help heal not just myself, but also other people on their journey through life.

In a strange way, I am infinitely grateful for my depression. I look back with appreciation to those black times: for in order to find the light, we sometimes need to work through the darkness. To this day, I still acknowledge the imbalances in my body: I shall be healing myself till the day I die. But not a day goes by without me affirming positively for what I want in my life. One of my favourite affirmations is this one:

"I love myself. I accept myself. I tune into the joy, happiness and laughter inside of me and share it outwardly."

I hope you enjoy this book as much as I enjoyed putting it together. If it helps just one person to overcome a health problem, then I shall know it is a success. Happy reading!

Breda.

Breda Gardner
Insight Natural Health Clinic
15 Upper Patrick St
Kilkenny
Tel: 056 7724429

Breda Gardner
Health Therapies Clinic
13 Gladstone St
Waterford
Tel: 051 858584

www.bredagardner.com

Email: breda@bredagardner.com

My website contains details of all my latest courses, events, meditation CD's and complementary health products, plus a page of useful addresses and links concerning complementary / natural health.

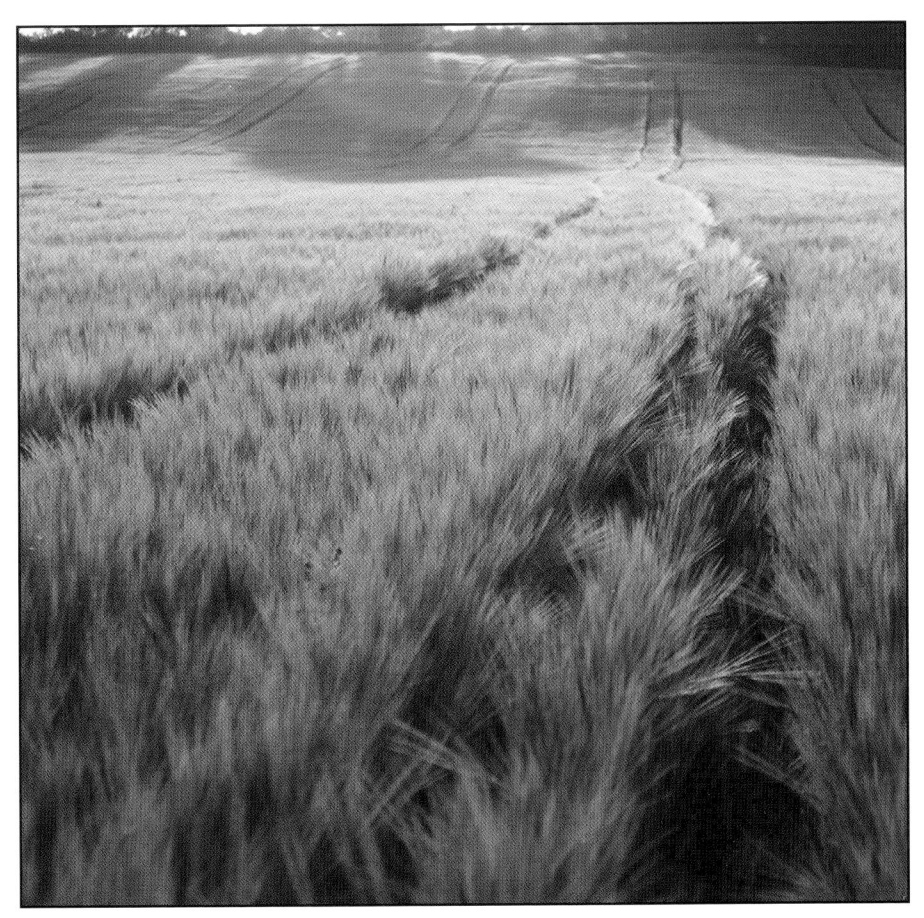

"We must always change, renew, rejuvenate ourselves; otherwise we harden."
~ Johann Wolfgang von Goethe

BEFORE YOU BEGIN!

Safety statement

Although my background is in conventional medicine – I qualified as a nurse in Jervis St, Dublin, and worked as a nurse for 15 years – many of the opinions expressed in this book do question some of the traditional tenets of conventional medicine. If you are in any doubt whatsoever about any of the topics covered in this book, you should consult a registered health professional. But don't be afraid to ask questions of your doctors. You might be surprised by their response: the article on antibiotics, for example, was verified with an eminent UK consultant. I also count a number of GP's amongst my clients. Remember that conventional medicine does not always have all the answers.

Advice on how to take homeopathic remedies

When I mention homeopathic remedies for acute situations (eg you have a thorn, or are suffering from shock), then I have included directions on how often to take them. For more chronic – or long term – conditions, I typically recommend that you take a 30 potency morning and evening for two weeks, and then take a break for two weeks to give your body the opportunity to heal. In either case, you should stop taking the dosage when the condition clears. If you would like to learn more about the healing properties of homeopathy, arrange a consultation with your local homeopath, or come along to my Homeopathic First Aid & Positive Living Course which I run twice a year, once in Kilkenny and once in Waterford.

A few other points to note:

Remember that homeopathic medicine includes conventional medicine too! So if you are prescribing remedies, remember simple first aid rules like keeping wounds clean, cooling burns under cold running water, reassuring the patient and so on!

Don't be afraid to experiment: if a remedy doesn't work, try another. It helps to keep a record of what you prescribe: soon you will build up a storehouse of information as to which remedies work best for you and your family.

Don't always expect an immediate reaction! Although some remedies – for example Arnica – can often give spectacular immediate results, others need more time to work.

Some remedies will make you worse before you get better. The remedy can zap the body's vital force, making you feel tired as healing takes place internally.

Above all, don't be afraid of homeopathic remedies: remember, they are safe, gentle and effective, and don't have side effects.

Homeopathic remedies are available from your health store, and increasingly, from pharmacists. Details of homeopathic pharmacies are given in the useful addresses section at the end of the book.

1
BODY / MIND RELATIONSHIPS

INTRODUCTION

Q: *I really enjoyed your articles on the different homeopathic personalities. You mentioned the relationship between the emotions and certain organs in the body. This is something that really fascinates me, and I was wondering if you could explain more on this topic.*

A: Thank you for your kind words. The link between our emotions and our bodies is a topic that never ceases to amaze me. In the olden, pre-scientific days, people were more connected to - and had more insight into - the specific link between emotions and the organs in the body. I believe that each person carries their own doctor inside them. But gone are the days when we used to heal ourselves with natural remedies and plenty of rest. We seem to have become powerless in our own bodies, and have lost contact with our own inner voice of intuition. We need to remember that science doesn't have all the answers, and that science is sometimes wrong – the recent Port Laoise breast scanning mistakes are a case in point. When we start to accept more responsibility for our own health, and when we tune into and listen to the symptoms in our body, a seemingly miraculous event takes place – we start to understand our feelings more, and we understand how they can and do influence our physical bodies.

I have some sympathy for GP's – it seems that many of their patients refuse to take any responsibility for their own health, and go to their GP to ask for a quick fix to the problem. They insist on playing the blame game – "I'm unwell because of my genes, or because I'm unhappy with my job or because I'm in an unhappy marriage" and so on. No! Often you are unwell because you choose to be unwell, consciously or unconsciously, and because you are so out of touch with your physical body, your emotions and your feelings. These patients only start to feel better once their GP has reassured them that everything is OK, that the tests are negative, and that they need to stop worrying. Only then do they feel better in themselves and do their physical symptoms start to disappear. In many cases, it can be mind over matter – if you believe that you can be healthy, then health comes your way. If you dwell on illness, illness comes your way.

Nowadays, people choose to live too much in their heads. They don't want to connect to their bodies, or are simply unaware of what is going on inside them.

But our physical complaints are talking to us and letting us know something is wrong. When we are ill, our bodies are saying "WAKE UP! LISTEN TO ME! I NEED MORE EMOTIONAL SUPPORT AND HELP!" But what do most people choose to do? They ignore their bodies, and suppress the problem with a painkiller, or with antibiotics or with steroids. Anything to take away the symptoms!

So hopefully, this series of articles will help you to establish a better relationship between your mind and your body. The simple act of bringing awareness to the part of ourselves that has been ignored is healing in itself. Every cell in our physical body is in constant communication with our thoughts, emotions, desires, beliefs and self-esteem.

The first stage of healing is understanding the inner conflict between the mind and body. The next step is transforming this relationship from a painful energy to a positive energy that enables healing to take place. So in these articles I will be writing about practical ways to enhance the healer inside of you. Don't live in denial or resistance, just acknowledge and let go – you will be amazed at the results!

BODY / MIND RELATIONSHIPS: BACK PAIN

From a body / mind relationship perspective, the back can be considered as the area where we store everything that we do not want to look at. This might manifest itself in a desire to run away from something or someone, or a wish to get things off our backs. The back is the support system of the body, so if you are suffering from back pains, it may mean that you are not feeling supported, be it in yourself or from the people around you.

Each part of the back represents different energies:

Upper back: this is the area behind the heart. Pain in this area may arise due to a lack of emotional support. You may feel unloved, or you may be holding back and not expressing love yourself. Many repressed and negative feelings may be stored in this part of the back. Try this affirmation to release the blockage / pain in this area: "I love myself. Life supports and loves me."

Middle back: the area where guilt is stored, where you worry about yourself or about others. Are you accepting yourself as you are? Are you too self-critical? Do you continually compare yourself to others? If so, this might be causing problems in your middle back. Try this affirmation: "I accept myself. I do my best at all times. I connect to the joy inside me."

Lower back: can represent resentment towards others. How often have you bent over backwards to accommodate someone, only for them to forget to acknowledge your help? Lower back pain can also arise from a great fear of moving forward, from a fear of not having enough money, or from a perceived lack of financial support. Try this affirmation: "I trust. I deserve abundance in my life. I am comfortable with my own power. I embrace change easily."

I am not suggesting for one minute that all back pain is caused by negative feelings, guilt or resentment. But what I am saying is that based on what I have learned from my clients over the past five years, I strongly believe two things: first that there is a definite link between what we think and certain areas of our bodies (like the connection between back pain and negative thoughts, guilt and resentment), and second that by using our minds positively, we can have a hugely beneficial effect on our health. So if you suffer from back pain, why not try one of the affirmations above? Affirm the words to yourself three times every morning and evening for two weeks, and believe in what you are saying. You have nothing to lose apart from your negative emotions, and best of all it's free to do!

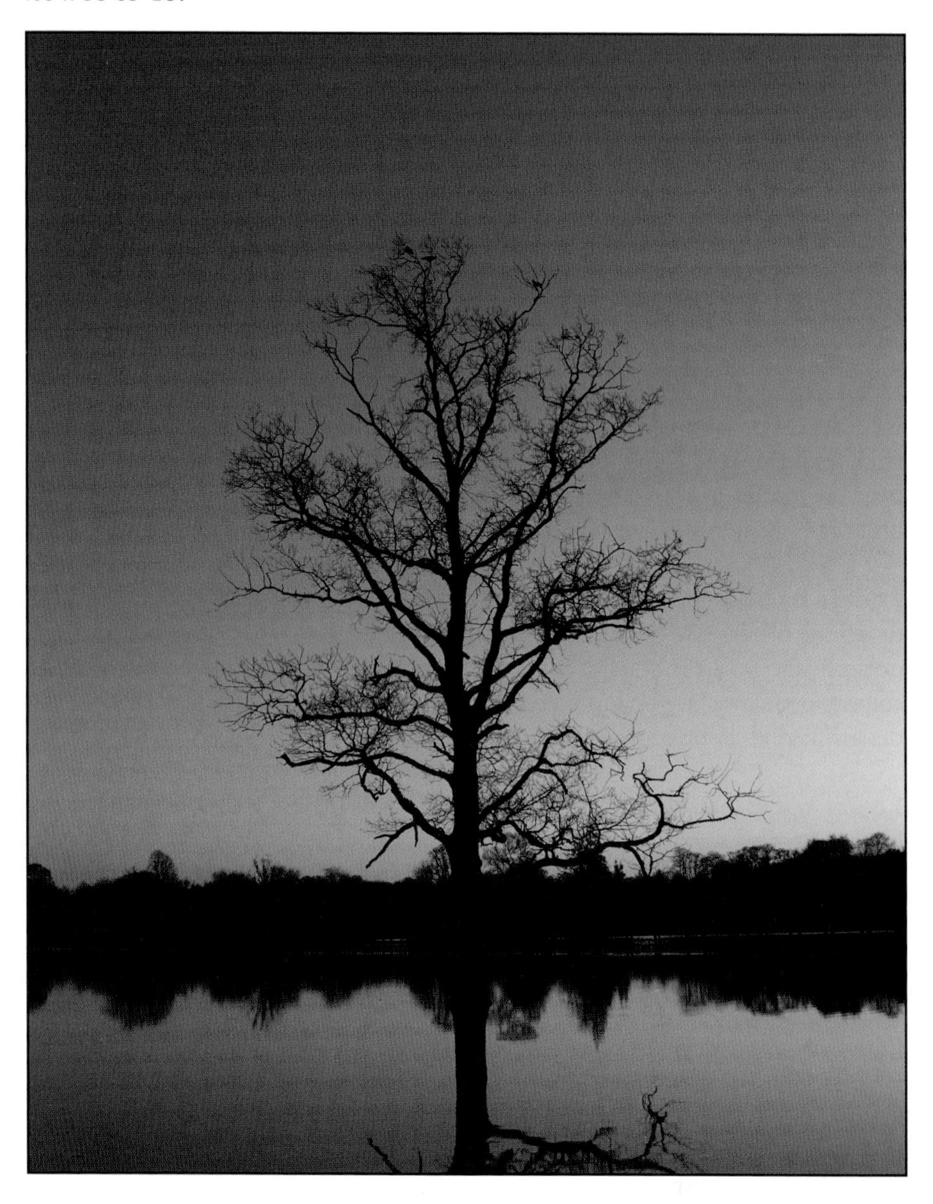

"Wisdom is knowing that silence often speaks louder than words."

BODY / MIND RELATIONSHIPS: THE BREASTS

For we women, our breasts represent our femininity, our relationship to ourselves, and our sexuality. Are we comfortable with being a woman? Are we taken seriously by our family, friends and colleagues? Or are we just seen as a sex symbol?

The breasts are the providers of nourishment and life, both in the form of food (breast-feeding) and in the form of comfort, reassurance and sexuality. However, if we as women are confused about ourselves, if we do not love ourselves enough, and if we fear rejection, then this can result in cysts, lumps or tender breasts. Women can also feel conflict from the outside world in their breasts. Such conflicts include rejection as a woman in a man's world! Women are expected to have children, and then either stay at home or work. But if a woman does not want to have children, is there something wrong with her? Is she any less of a woman?

Breast cancer in women may indicate deep mental thought patterns, sometimes engrained since childhood, with a deep hurt, resentment or silent grief eating away at the self. (As an aside, in men, breast cancer can be connected to feelings of self worth, about a desire to be accepted and an inability to express the feminine aspect of caring and nurturing inherent in all human beings, male and female.)

Having healthy breasts means allowing your full womanhood to emerge. This does not mean you have to be a mother, or have perfect breasts. It means allowing the deepest qualities of wisdom, intuition, love and compassion to emerge from within. It means accepting yourself as you are, and knowing that your inner qualities are far superior to the outside views held by society at large. Keep loving yourself and allow others to be who they are. Know that you are safe in this world and that self-love is the key to self-healing.

I see many women in my clinics who suffer from breast tenderness. Many assume that it is normal to have these symptoms, as they have had them for years. I recommend that they try the homeopathic remedy Pulsatilla 30 potency morning and evening for two weeks to help balance the lymphatic system and hence reduce the tenderness. Cutting out all dairy products (that includes milk, cheese and chocolate) also helps the circulatory lymphatic system to work more efficiently.

BODY / MIND RELATIONSHIPS: THE HEART

The heart is associated with love and represents the very core of our emotions. It is the centre of our passion, and, on a higher level, our compassion. Our hearts are connected to a whole range of feelings, from love, compassion and tenderness, to grief, loss, fear and guilt. "He stole my heart away … She broke my heart … My heart's one desire … In my heart of hearts I knew … I let my heart rule my head …" – all these phrases illustrate and reinforce the role and importance of the heart in our feelings.

We can quite literally feel pain in our heart when it is broken – indeed people can die from a broken heart. In times of stress or unhappiness, it can seem like a set of armour is tightening around the chest and heart. But the opposite is true too – when our hearts are joyful, we experience a wonderful and unequalled sense of expansion and energy that makes us feel lighter in ourselves – just remember how you felt the first time you fell in love!

Heart attacks may occur where joy has been squeezed out of the body. A person who worries too much about what they don't have or should have - instead of accepting what they already have – may suffer from a build-up in cholesterol in the body. Worrying too much creates anxiety, causing the heart to palpitate. It is important to learn to breathe slowly and deeply in everyday living. This helps the heart to relax, making the blood flow around the body more efficiently and effectively.

The emotion guilt can also be detrimental to the heart and its energy. Guilt places pressure on the heart. Why carry extra weight on yourself by connecting to guilt? All the heart really wants to do is to connect to joy and fun, and by doing this, you help to alkalise the body and dissolve cholesterol.

When our hearts and emotions are balanced, we feel unrestrained joy. This can give us the most tremendous feeling for beauty, for music, for poetry and so on. This joy radiates out from us and on to those around us, guiding us to the world of love. So use your heart wisely: keep loving yourself first, then give your love unconditionally, and watch the rewards come back into your life. The following affirmation may also be of assistance: say it to yourself 20 times morning and evening for two weeks:

"I tune into the love, joy, happiness and laughter within my heart, and share them all outwardly."

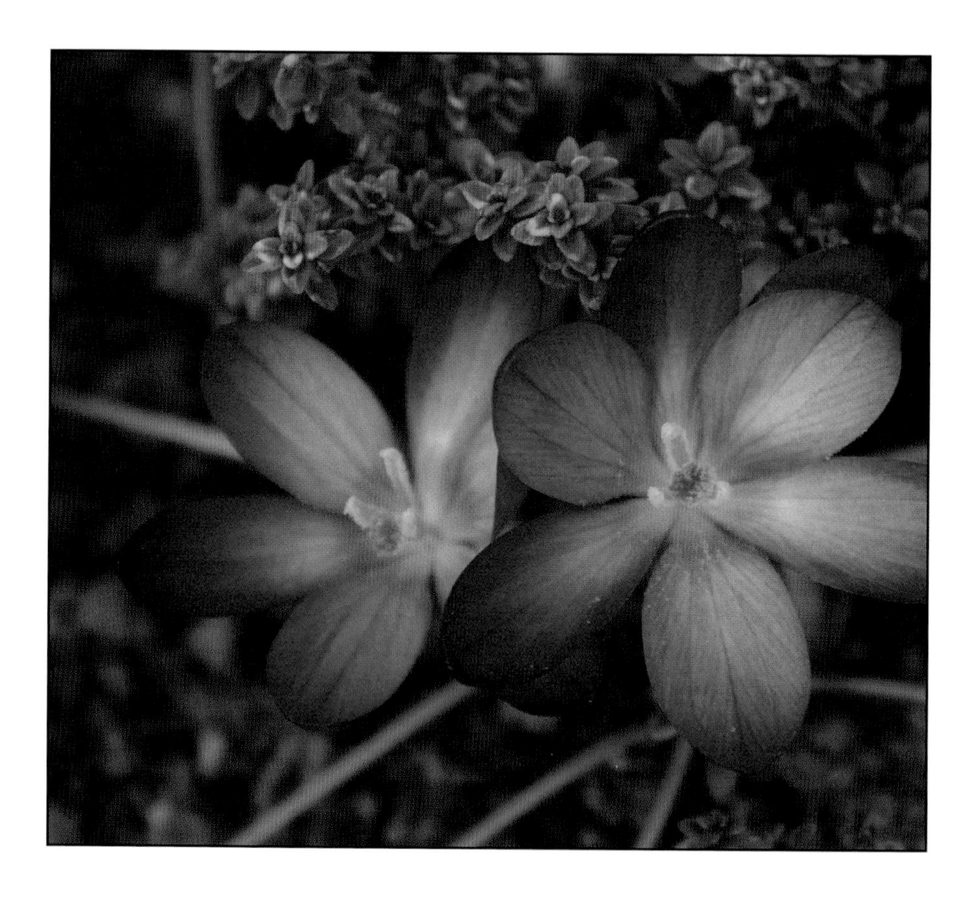

"A loving heart is the truest wisdom. " ~ *Charles Dickens*

BODY / MIND RELATIONSHIPS: THE KIDNEYS & BLADDER

The primary role of the kidneys is to filter impurities from the blood and to pass on these impurities to the bladder. The bladder acts as a chamber for holding these waste impurities before releasing them in urine. So from a body / mind perspective, these organs are mainly connected to the cleansing and releasing of negative emotions held in the body. Our emotions are mainly concerned with relationships – relationships with ourselves, with others and with the world we live in. When the energy around the kidneys and bladder is good, we are able to stand on our own two feet, feel comfortable in our own skin, and are less dependent on other people.

In my experience, fear is often stored in the unconscious cellular memory of the kidneys and bladder – a fear of expression, of self-survival, of relationships, of death and so on. If such fear is present in the body, it may express itself in a wide range of physical symptoms such as panic attacks, feelings of nervousness (worse for loud noises), repeated cystitis (with feelings of ultra sensitivity), heart palpitations, vertigo and dizzy spells, headaches, a feeling of choking on swallowing, heart attacks, chest infections and angina. Many of these symptoms may feel as though they are coming from the stomach.

The bladder helps to release our negative emotions in the urine and to stop us from drowning in our own negativity. Anxiety can be stored in the bladder – a fear of letting go, or just being "peed off" with life. This may come out in the body as cystitis. Cystitis is an infection of the urinary system, and can be viewed as a means of releasing emotions that are no longer needed.

Excess tea can weaken the kidneys and bladder, because the tannin in tea can dehydrate the body. My advice is to limit your intake to 2 cups of tea daily, to drink more filtered water, and to try herbal teas which are more alkaline and hydrating for the body (regular tea, like coffee, is acidic).

The homeopathic remedy Aconite can help to release fear stored in the kidneys and bladder. Try a 30 potency morning and evening for two weeks only, and then give the body time to heal itself. You can also try the following affirmation - say it to yourself 20 times morning and evening for two weeks:

"It is safe to be me. I enjoy life. I let go of the past and embrace the present. I love me."

BODY / MIND RELATIONSHIPS: THE LIVER

After the skin, the liver is the second largest organ in the body. It absorbs and stores fats and proteins, as well as helping to maintain the sugar level in the blood. The liver also helps to detox poisons that enter the body, and plays an important role in our immune system.

From a body / mind perspective, the liver stores and processes the emotion of "anger" – by removing anger from the blood, it helps to keep us emotionally balanced. When it is functioning well, the liver ensures we wake up energised and feel ready and motivated to get on with the challenges in the day ahead – we say "Good morning, God!" But if the energy of the liver is poor, we wake up feeling tired, apathetic and sluggish, saying "Good God it's morning!"

Anger which goes inwards can lead to depression. So ask yourself whether you harbour any bitter, resentful thoughts or feelings that are not being expressed or resolved. One of my clients once said to me "If only I could get angry, then I wouldn't feel so helpless in myself." He found it hard to express his anger, so he kept his negative thoughts to himself and thus felt disempowered. I advised him to exercise more, to help channel his energy better. I also advised him that when he was in his car or at home on his own, he should scream as loud as he could, just to help release his blocked energy. He subsequently told me that he followed this advice, and screamed out loud when he was out walking in a forest on his own … only to turn the corner and meet a shocked couple coming the other way! So you might want to take care where you follow this suggestion! My client did say, however, that he felt 100% better for letting his anger out.

I often think it would be a good idea if every workplace had a padded, insulated room where employees could go to let off steam. I'm sure that we've all been in a situation at work where we could happily have walked into such a place and screamed at the top of our voices and punched the padded wall! I could almost guarantee that if such a room existed in our offices and factories, there would be less sickness and more happiness within the workplace!

The liver's role in the immune system emphasises how influential negative thoughts and feelings can affect our general state of health. When there is a block in the liver energy, you may feel very indecisive, crave sweet things, become angry easily, or simply feel angry inside, with feelings of apathy, no motivation, and a general sense of insecurity about yourself. You may feel very stuck, like you are not getting anywhere. You may also find yourself always worrying about the future, and feel that you lack a sense of purpose or direction in your life.

The homeopathic remedy Lycopodium can help to get a sluggish liver moving again. Take a 30 potency morning and evening for two weeks only. Repeat one month later if needed. Lycopodium helps to detox the liver and make you think more positive thoughts. You can also try the following affirmation – say it to yourself 20 times morning and evening for two weeks and see if it makes a difference:

"I trust. I embrace change easily. I think positive thoughts always. I connect to the peace within me. All is well in my world."

BODY / MIND RELATIONSHIPS: THE SKIN

The skin is the largest organ in the body. It is made up of soft tissue, and corresponds directly to our mental energy, our past experiences, our attitudes and our patterns of behaviour. Traumas and conflicts can be buried deep in the soft tissues of our skin.

In my experience, skin problems often mean that a person's individuality is being threatened. It may be that you feel powerless and thin-skinned – things literally get under your skin and irritate you. Are you holding on to old hurts and disappointments? Do you feel let down? Can you forgive easily? Are you so sensitive that you isolate yourself from your own feelings and other people, so that you will not get hurt again? Psoriasis can result from a fear of being hurt and a refusal to accept responsibility for our own feelings.

It may be that you are thick-skinned and nothing can get through to you. Are you stubborn and obstinate towards both yourself and others? Do you always have to have an opinion on everything – and is your opinion always right? (and no-one will ever change it!). If you are thick-skinned, this can create an excess of mental energy that can block the energy flow to the rest of your body and hence lead to a skin reaction.

Or perhaps you feel skinned alive? You feel hard done by, that your power has been taken away, and that you are a victim, full of resentment and anger. If resentment builds up in the blood and anger in the liver, an outlet is needed to protect the other inner organs – and that outlet often overflows into the skin, creating skin disorders.

Any skin irritation can indicate a general irritation or frustration with what you are doing - or what you are not doing! We blush with embarrassment, we redden with anger or go white with fear as the skin constantly reflects our feelings.

If you are suffering from a skin complaint, the following affirmation can be of help. Try to say it 20 times twice daily to encourage more positive thought patterns, and to get more positive energy flowing through your body:

"I forgive easily. I feel safe and secure. I take responsibility for myself. I empower myself easily. I embrace change effortlessly. I trust that everything is OK."

As ever, it is also important to drink 8 to 10 glasses of filtered water a day to help hydrate the skin and body.

BODY / MIND RELATIONSHIPS: THE STOMACH

The stomach's role is to break down food so that it can be easily absorbed. It is also the area where we take in, assimilate and digest our reality – we extract what is wanted and eliminate what is not needed. Thus the stomach is where we hold on to – or let go of – personal issues. The stomach is emotionally linked to love (of the self and for others), to food and to your relationship with your mother!

You may have heard the phrases "I can't stomach what's going on around me" or "You are not what you eat, but what you assimilate." Both phrases indicate that if you are unhappy, very sensitive or take things too personally, then this can affect your digestion, and lead to real physical symptoms like heartburn, constant burping, nausea and butterflies in the stomach. Conversely, if you are happy and you feel healthy, your food is broken down easily and is readily absorbed.

Food can spend many hours in the stomach before being absorbed, so it is not too surprising to find that your thoughts and feelings can also sit in this area. If your thoughts are negative, tension may be felt in the stomach area, and this can lead to digestive problems. The stomach is linked to a centre of energy called the solar plexus, which in turn is concerned with whether we are liked or disliked, and whether we have power or not. This is where we hold our fears and insecurities or become obsessed with thinking of ourselves as the greatest and most successful. It can be a centre of egotism where there is an inability to share with others and therefore meaning we have no peace within ourselves.

Food is eaten for survival ("you should eat to live, not live to eat!" as the saying goes), but food can also represent mother, love, security, happiness and reward. Eating sweet food is a way of feeding ourselves the sweetness or reward that we may feel nobody else is giving us. Food can be used as a great comfort.

The stomach can talk to us in many ways. One example is that if you are not comfortable with your own power and feel used, then you may have the sensation of butterflies fluttering in your stomach. Another example is a client I saw who was four stone overweight. She told me that her mother kept harassing her to lose weight. She was very hurt by her mother's accusations and felt they were like a knife to the stomach. So when she returned home that evening after the accusations, she dug in relentlessly into the fridge, and ate lots of ice cream until she felt sick. This lack of love for herself stopped her from standing up for herself. I advised her to ask her mother to respect her feelings and to not speak down to her: if her mother had done so, then my client might not have gone home and eaten all the ice cream!

I see many clients who are very sensitive: they take things far too personally, make assumptions that are not true, and let other people walk all over them. Such clients often suffer from gastritis, heartburn or ulcers.

So if any of the above sounds like you, then here are some steps you can take to help strengthen your stomach:

- **See mealtimes as a sacred time to enjoy and digest your food. Make time to sit and chew - and enjoy! - your food slowly (30 – 40 bites per mouthful of food). Digestion starts in the mouth with saliva, which eases the work of the stomach.**
- **Don't drink with meals – wait until 15 – 20 minutes before and after eating, so the hydrochloric acid in your stomach can break down your food more easily. If you must drink, take only small sips. Try drinking meadowsweet tea before or after meals - it balances the hydrochloric acid and aids digestion.**
- **Don't eat if you are very anxious, worried or nervous – try and relax first, go for a walk in nature and take deep breaths to help relax your body.**
- **Apple cider vinegar (try a tablespoon mixed with a little water and honey) is a popular drink to alkalise the stomach and help improve digestion.**

The homeopathic remedies Nat Mur, Nux Vomica and Pulsatilla can also be of assistance. Nat Mur makes your stomach assimilate your food better, and helps you to detach from emotional arguments. Nux Vomica relaxes the stomach as well as helping you to be less anxious, and to live more in the now and less in the head. Pulsatilla is excellent if you have a bloated stomach with indigestion. It helps you to stand up for yourself, and eases the transition from low energy foods (like ice cream, biscuits and cakes etc) to high energy foods (like salads, fruits, brown rice etc).

You can also try the following affirmations – say them to yourself as often as possible for two weeks:

"I embrace the now. I assimilate my food and enjoy life more."

"I love myself and empower myself easily."

2
WHAT IS MAKING ME ILL?

INTRODUCTION

Have you ever thought about what makes us ill? I don't mean viruses or bacteria or parasites, but rather the things that can disrupt the balance in our bodies and make us susceptible to disease.

In my clinics, I like to use something called the circle of health to illustrate how a wide range of factors can influence our health. When the circle of health is strong and unbroken, people's energy levels are good, and they can cope with the stresses and strains that come their way. They feel at peace with themselves, have no anger, and live in the now, being happy and gracious for what they have, and giving out love. They have no fear of the future, and trust becomes part of their everyday life. This allows them to be less controlling and brings synchronicity into their lives.

But when there are cracks in the circle, then the body may go out of balance, with symptoms like fatigue, migraine, hormonal imbalances, depression, heart problems, gastric and skin disorders and so on: the list is endless!

So what causes the cracks in the circle of health? How can we identify them, and how can we fix them? The answer to the first question is that there are many potential causes, including:

1. Dehydration
2. Electromagnetic stress
3. Geopathic stress
4. Mercury toxicity
5. Metal toxicity
6. Chemical toxicity
7. Poor nutrition
8. Fears
9. Anger
10. Loss & Sadness
11. Guilt & Shame
12. Constitutional & genetic weaknesses.

To help identify the cracks in the circle, I use a combination of my medical knowledge from many years of nursing, iridology (reading the irises of the eyes), muscle testing and listening carefully to what my clients are saying. And to help fix the cracks, I use homeopathy, positive affirmations, flower essences and advice on nutrition.

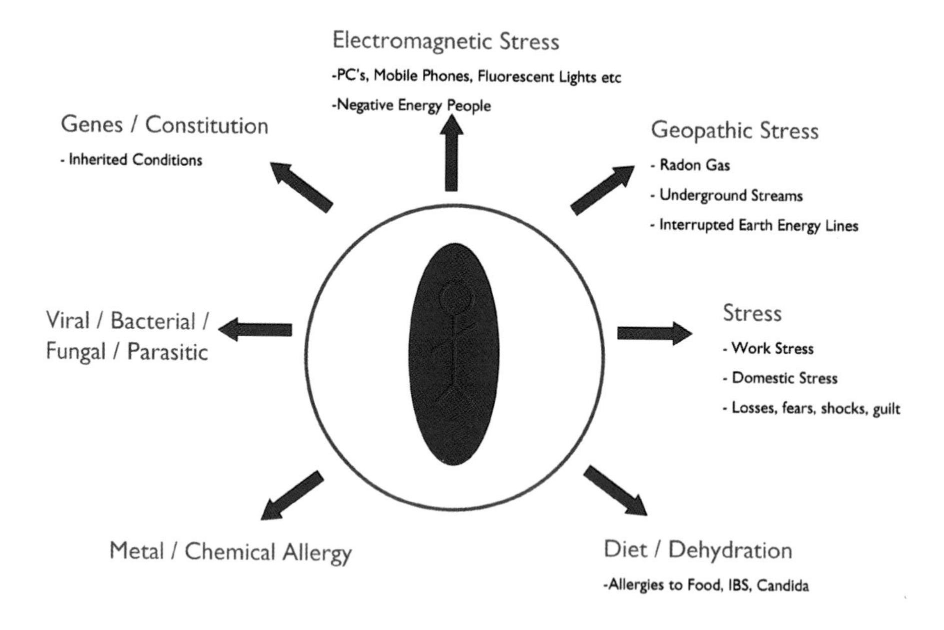

The Circle of Health

THE HEALING POWER OF WATER

Like the sun, water is a basic necessity of life. In my clinics, one of the first things I test for is dehydration in my clients. My first prescription is to drink filtered water. Everybody assumes that they drink enough water, but coffee, tea, fizzy drinks and alcohol all dehydrate the body. If you drink 3 cups of coffee daily and 3 good-sized glasses of water, then you are still at zero positive hydration. Moreover, excess coffee and alcohol can damage the liver, and excess tea may weaken the kidneys. So my advice is to cut back to no more than 2 cups of tea or coffee a day, and to drink 8 – 10 glasses of water a day. In the morning, instead of tea or coffee, try squeezing half a lemon into boiled water to help detox your system: you can add a spoonful of manuka honey if you don't like the taste!

A lack of water prevents our bodies from flourishing: it can cause our health to deteriorate and our ageing to accelerate. Most of us suffer from insufficient water and "dry out" as the years go by. Dry skin, cracked lips and stiff joints are often outward signs of a lack of water, yet we usually attribute these obvious signs of dehydration and a lack of lubrication to some other cause.

Our bodies consist of 60 - 70% water. Without water, the cells in our bodies cannot function, nor can we digest and eliminate our foods so easily. Plenty of water helps to dilute the toxins in our bodies, to stop constipation, and to lessen the possibility of urinary infections. Finally, our brains are around 80% water, which explains why dehydration can lead to poor memory.

Remember that to keep our body fluids balanced, we need about 4 pints of water each day. The need will vary with each individual. A diet high in fruit and salad may provide up to 1.5 to 2 pints daily, and other beverages, eg freshly squeezed juices, may provide up to a pint. But if you drink tea, coffee, cocoa or alcohol, or if you use diuretic drugs or salt, then your need for water will be higher. Water is the cheapest medicine for the body, keeping your cells cleansed and healthy. Drink water and stay healthy!

ELECTROMAGNETIC STRESS - PART 1

Q: *I recently attended one of your empowerment workshops, and found it very enlightening. You spoke briefly on how and why the body can become ill from electromagnetic stress. I found this subject fascinating, and was wondering of you could explain further.*

A:Thanks for your kind words, and I'm glad you enjoyed the workshop. There are many maintaining causes as to why the body goes out of balance, and one of them is electromagnetic stress (EMS). I define electromagnetic stress as negative energy that affects the body. This negative energy can take many forms, such as excess radiation from computer screens, mobile phones, games consoles, pylons, cars, fluorescent lights and other similar electric / electronic devices. But EMS can also be caused by our own negative thoughts (living too much in the head), and by bad vibrations from negative people.

In our bodies, we have an area called the solar plexus. The solar plexus (the breast bone) is positioned between the top of the stomach and the base of the lungs. When we are stressed out, or when we are susceptible to EMS, the solar plexus is often the part of the body which is most affected. Symptoms of EMS may include constant fatigue, dizziness, headaches and migraines, a general lack of energy and vitality, insomnia, poor concentration, hyperactivity, gastritis and a general tendency to over-react to situations or to be very impulsive. EMS can also lower your immune system, allowing other viruses / bacteria to multiply, and leading to illness in the weakest organs in the body. In my clinics, I use a simple technique called muscle testing to help diagnose EMS in the body.

In Part 1, I will cover EMS caused by excessive exposure to electromagnetic radiation, and in Part 2, I will say more on how negative energy and negative people can and do affect our health.

One of the many symptoms of EMS in the body is static shocks: if you have ever touched your car door and received a shock, you will know exactly what I'm talking about! Alternatively, have you ever sat in front of a computer screen for hours at a time, and by the end of the day you feel utterly exhausted? In both cases, I believe these symptoms are a reminder to let you know that you are stressed out, living too much in your head, and are – quite literally - not grounded.

As a demonstration of the unhealthy effects of EMS, I once saw a teenage girl who for months had been suffering from sleep problems and constant headaches. She had had repeated CAT scans which came back NAD (no abnormality detected), but her symptoms persisted. On diagnosis, I found that she was suffering from EMS, and on further questioning I discovered that she used to sleep with her mobile phone under her pillow. I advised her to immediately desist from doing this, and to use a magnetic wave shield on her phone. By doing these two things, she removed the maintaining cause of her sleeplessness and headaches, and I was delighted to learn on her next visit that her symptoms had disappeared. I see many people in my clinics who are extremely sensitive to – and suffer from – EMS like this, but once the maintaining cause is identified and removed, clients have had excellent results.

Excess radiation can enter the body via the ear (as in the case described above), or via the solar plexus which is often at the same level as the source of radiation, eg a computer screen. Our body's energies should flow from head to toe, hence static shocks can be there to remind us that we are not grounded enough in our lives. So if this sounds like you, what can you do to lessen the effects of EMS? Here are some suggestions:

- **Remove all electrics from your bedside, ie lamps, electric clocks / blankets, hifis, TV's etc. They should be at least three feet away from you, otherwise they can affect your own energy field.**
- **Use a magnetic wave shield on devices like mobile phones, Nintendo DS's etc (I recommend the "Waveshield" brand of magnetic protectors, which have been scientifically proven to reduce the amount of electromagnetic radiation that may enter through the inner ear).**
- **Use deep breathing exercises, positive affirmations and meditation to ground yourself.**
- **Take homeopathic remedies to help boost the immune system and balance the body (consult with your local homeopath).**
- **Take a break! - don't spend too long in front of the screen, on the phone or playing a game.**
- **If you sit in front of a computer all day long, place a black tourmaline crystal in front of your screen to help absorb radiation and protect you (it's important that you rinse the crystal under running water every few weeks to maintain its effectiveness).**

- **If you live near a pylon or mobile phone mast, black tourmaline crystals can also help to reduce the negative energy.**

If you are interested, you can purchase Waveshield EMS radiation protectors and black tourmaline crystals at either of my clinics in Kilkenny and Waterford.

ELECTROMAGNETIC STRESS – PART 2

In Part 1, I wrote about the potentially harmful effects of electromagnetic stress (EMS) caused by man-made electrical devices like mobile phones, computers, playstations etc. In this article I'm covering the EMS caused by negative people or negative thoughts.

Suppose you meet someone at work or on the street and they assume that you have done them wrong. They insult you angrily, yet you have no idea where their anger has come from. Do you take it personally - in other words eat the poison apple? If you do take it personally, you have let their negative energy inside your body. This can affect your body's cells and bring on unwanted thoughts in your head, which turn around like a hamster on a wheel. In due course this can bring on physical ailments like stomach problems, headaches or backaches.

Nelson Mandela is a wonderful example of a man upon whom injustice was heaped, having spent 27 years in prison as an innocent man. He came out of prison an enlightened man and not at all bitter. He managed to detach himself from his situation, saying "Why should I be bitter? My captors were only doing what they felt was right for them at the time."

Question: Why can't we all be more like Nelson Mandela? Answer: because we eat other people's emotional garbage, and then it becomes ours. When we take things personally, we feel offended, we over-react to defend our beliefs, and hence create conflicts. We make a mountain out of a molehill, because we have a need to be in the right. If you are an enlightened person with positive energy, you accept yourself as you are, and you do not need the approval of other people. In addition, you stop taking on other people's negative energy, and just accept that it is their opinions that have created their own conflicts.

Everyone's point of view is something personal to them. If you get mad at someone, know that you are dealing with yourself and your own issues. You get mad because you are afraid and you have to face your own fears. If you love yourself, there is no place for any of these negative, fearful emotions.

So whatever people do, feel, think or say, the first rule is not to take it personally. Just radiate love inwardly and outwardly to eliminate EMS from your body.

When we see other people as they really are, without taking things personally, we can never be hurt by what they say or do. Your anger, jealousy, envy and even your sadness will disappear. Try to detach yourself from your emotions and look back in on the situation from a positive viewpoint.

Where clients are suffering from negative people or from their own negative thoughts, I advise them to use positive affirmations every morning and evening, and also to improve their diet and lifestyle choices – for example, more fresh fruit and vegetables, less coffee and tea, more walks in nature, and more time doing the things you enjoy, like singing, dancing, gardening or whatever it is that makes you happy. To combat negative people, I encourage my clients to believe "What you think of me is none of my business!" Be happy, be positive, stop taking things too personally, don't always be making assumptions, and remain connected to the now at all times. This will enhance your energy, making it flow better through your body, and helping to keep ill-health at bay. Certain homeopathic remedies can also help boost the immune system and balance the body in cases of EMS caused by negative thoughts or negative people (see your local homeopath for more information).

This simple exercise can also help to ensure you maintain positive energy in your body:

Breathe in deeply through your nose to the count of 1 … 2 … 3. Hold for a second and exhale slowly though your mouth, using the lips like a valve. As you inhale, say to yourself, "I am breathing in positive energy, I am breathing in joy, happiness and peace." As you exhale, say to yourself, "I am breathing out negative energy, I am breathing out all my tensions, worries, fears and sadness." Try this exercise for five minutes every morning and evening, and I guarantee that you will feel more empowered and balanced in yourself. Go on – try the exercise for a few weeks, and feel the difference in your life and energy levels!

GEOPATHIC STRESS

Have you ever been in a house, office or place outdoors which makes you feel uneasy? If so, you may have been picking up on geopathic stress. Geopathic literally means "suffering from the earth", and geopathic stress can result from factors like the excessive emission of radon gas, or from the magnetic disturbance caused by the confluence of two underground streams. When narrow paths of water converge - sometimes as much as 200 or 300 feet below the ground - they can create an electromagnetic field which distorts the earth's natural vibrations as they pass through the water. Certain mineral concentrations, fault lines, moving underground plateaus and underground cavities can also disturb the earth's natural vibrations. The Chinese art of "Feng Shui" places great importance on the balancing of these disturbances of the earth's vibrations.

Dowsers and diviners can detect geopathic stress in a house or premises: in my clinics, I use a simple muscle testing technique with a vial of geopathic stress to detect it in people.

Geopathic stress can have a strong effect on the lymphatic system. The lymph fluid transports lymphocytes and antibodies which fight and destroy any foreign cells in the body, such as bacteria, viruses or cancer cells. If the lymphatic system is not healthy, then it may have difficulty in destroying foreign bodies, including cancer cells, thus allowing them to grow and multiply. Your whole immune system can become weakened. Symptoms of geopathic stress include:

- **Fatigue and feeling run down**
- **Restless sleep and insomnia**
- **Lack of appetite**
- **Muscular cramps or increased heartbeat, especially in bed**
- **Depression and nervousness**
- **Muffy head or sluggish on awakening in the morning**
- **When away from home, you sleep better and wake up fresher.**

Much research has been done on geopathic stress, and some of the findings are most interesting. It is estimated that more than 4,000 medical doctors in

Austria and Germany call in dowsers to assist with their most severe cases of cancer and long term illnesses. In many parts of Europe, it is commonplace for sites to be tested for geopathic stress before any building work begins. In Ireland, for example, building regulations require that every new house incorporates some degree of preventive measures against radon gas at the time of construction.

A study of the health of the travelling community also provided more intriguing results. Some 250 families took part in the study, and the conclusion was that cancer is a disease that is almost unknown to many traveller families, even when they ignored all the warnings about smoking, drinking and eating the wrong foods. One reason put forward is that they rarely stay in one place for a long time, and hence are not prone to the effects of geopathic stress.

So what can you do if you think you are suffering from geopathic stress? If you wish to have your house tested, then check out your local health store for the name of a reputable dowser. Otherwise you could try moving your bed to another part of your bedroom, or if there is not enough space, try clearing out the clutter from under your bed, and place rose quartz crystals there instead. All this will help to protect you from harmful, negative earth rays. It is important to wash the rose quartz under running water every month and then leave it in daylight for 12 hours to recharge it. Rose quartz has an amazing ability to help heal the heart energy. By healing your heart energy, you will find that you can give and receive love more easily. This in turn has a positive effect on your lymphatic system raising your immunity levels.

If you are worried about radon gas, you can contact the Radiological Protection Institute of Ireland (RPII) on 01 269 77 66, or see www.rpii.ie. The website has details of companies that offer a radon gas measurement service.

MERCURY TOXICITY

There has been much controversy over the effects of mercury fillings. So just what are the facts? Dental "amalgam" fillings are the silver-black coloured ones in most people's mouths. The amalgam typically consists of one half mercury, combined with silver, tin and other metals. Opponents of amalgam fillings claim that the mercury leaks continuously into the body's tissues, seriously affecting the person's health. Mercury has been linked to many illnesses, including allergies, Alzheimer's, angina, cancer, candida, chronic fatigue syndrome, depression, hypertension, multiple sclerosis, Parkinson's disease and psoriasis – the list goes on! In addition, many of us are exposed to mercury via our mother's fillings, coal smoke, industrial pollution, and certain medications and vaccinations.

A report sponsored by the World Health Organisation and United Nations concluded that (a) the use of mercury in amalgam silver fillings is hazardous to both human health and the environment (it is illegal to dispose of waste amalgam into the sewerage system), and (b) mercury fillings constitute the main mercury exposure risk to humans, exceeding food, air and water sources combined. The Swedish Parliament voted for a ban on amalgam as far back as 1994. In the USA, the first ban has also been passed. Since January 1st 2007, amalgam filling placements have been completely banned by the State of California.

So what can you do? There are a number of options. You can leave your existing mercury fillings where they are, and ask your dentist to use non-mercury fillings in the future. Or you can ask your dentist to replace your existing fillings, although there is a risk that removing them may lead to greater toxicity entering the blood system. You may have to choose a dentist who specialises in replacing amalgam fillings: for more information on such dentists in Ireland or Northern Ireland, contact the British Society for Mercury-Free Dentistry, PO Box 42606, London, SW5 0XA, UK, call 00 44 20 8746 1177, or go to www.mercuryfreedentistry.org.uk.

The homeopathic remedies Mercury and Spirulina can help to cleanse the blood if you feel you are suffering from the side effects of mercury toxicity (symptoms include increased salivation, recurrent mouth ulcers, bad breath and dark rings under the eyes). I usually use a simple kinesiology (muscle-testing) technique to find if mercury toxicity is a priority for treatment. I then use several detox homeopathic remedies to help build up the client's immune system. Hydrating your body with filtered water at all times is also helpful in reducing the toxicity.

I myself have had all my mercury fillings replaced with white fillings – I have had them now for over ten years with little or no ill effects. I strongly recommend changing your mercury fillings if it is a prime maintaining cause of your illness. But remember that you need to cut out sugar too – there in no point in having gleaming white teeth if the acid from sugar causes decay!

METAL TOXICITY

Have you ever worn a cheap pair of ear-rings which caused a rash on your ear? Or worn a watch which left a green deposit on your wrist? If so, then you have suffered from an allergy to metal. The examples just given are not too serious: you can avoid the problem by not wearing the ear-rings and watch. But metal allergies can be the cause of much more serious complaints.

Whilst gaining clinical experience in London some years ago, I recall seeing a young man in his 30's who had suffered from repeated urinary tract infections. He had been seeing a consultant in Harley Street for over three years with no success. Amazingly, he had been prescribed no less than 30 courses of antibiotics over this period. He was in constant pain, and nothing medically was helping him. My colleague in the clinic used diagnostic kinesiology (muscle-testing) and found him to be allergic to metal. It turned out that his wife had given him a silver watch for his birthday some four years previously, and that all his problems had begun about a year after that. Metal toxicity often has an affinity to deposit itself in the prostate gland or bladder, which was what was happening with this patient. He was told to remove his watch, to hydrate his body, and to take homeopathic medicine to strengthen the kidney/bladder area and to help detox the metal from his body. He made a speedy recovery once the maintaining cause – ie his watch – was removed.

Metal toxicity also has an affinity to affect the spine. If you have back trouble, try removing all metals from your body, and you may find you become less susceptible to aches and pains. My husband used to suffer repeatedly from a bad back, but since he stopped wearing a silver ring and a silver chain with a St Christopher medal, he has not had a problem.

Apart from jewellery and watches, there are several other potential causes of allergy from metals in contact with the body, such as spectacles, fillings, braces, fracture pins and other medical devices. The simplest way to avoid metal allergies is to avoid metals on your skin in the first place! If you do wear jewellery, try and choose the best quality you can. Gold is the best option: in its purest form it is hypoallergenic, ie it does not cause allergy, and it does not affect the skin, since it is a natural metal. Silver usually contains a mixture of nickel and other metals to which some people are highly intolerant. It is also crucial to keep your body hydrated: you may be allergic to metals, but if your body is sufficiently hydrated, then you may find there are no problems.

My own findings in my clinics are that people who are intolerant to metal appear to be more susceptible to candida (overgrowth of yeast). The metallic toxins seep in through the skin and travel around the body via the lymphatic system, depositing themselves either in the womb in women, or in the prostate gland / bladder in men.

CHEMICAL TOXICITY

The level of chemicals and pollutants that we are exposed to is at an all time high. When we think of harmful chemicals, most of us think of a smoggy, polluted, urban area. Unfortunately, many of the harmful toxins can be found in our own homes, and because of regular proximity to them, they can potentially do more harm than the smoke-belching factory!

Now I'm not suggesting for one moment that we are all sitting on deadly time bombs and are in mortal danger, but the fact remains that there are a number of dangerous toxins in our homes. The most obvious is cigarette smoke, not just for the smoker him or herself, but for the passive smokers too (second-hand tobacco smoke contains over 4,000 chemicals, many of which are carcinogenic). Our food and drink can be polluted: hormones and anti-biotics in meat, pesticides in vegetables and phenylalanine in orange squash. Many beauty products – like body creams and tanning lotions - also contain potentially harmful chemicals that can compromise our immune systems and hence form a barrier to health recovery. And finally, many of the cleaning and gardening products we use contain toxins.

A bad reaction to the chemicals in our lives can cause allergies, asthma, skin disorders, and even life-threatening conditions like cancer. So what can we do to help reduce the effects of these toxins? Whilst it is impossible to avoid all harmful chemicals in our day-to-day lives, it is relatively easy to dramatically reduce your exposure by simply paying more attention to the products that you use in your household, garden and on your body. It may involve a clear-out of your shelves and cupboards, but the benefits will be repaid by an ever greater surge in your health recovery. Here are some other tips:

- **Remove tobacco smoke from your home. If any of your family or friends smoke, they are free to do so ... outside!**
- **Clear out your usual domestic cleaning products and try healthier cleaning alternatives such as vinegar and water for windows, lemon juice for dishes and bathroom areas, baking powder and water for ovens. Undiluted white vinegar can be used as a household disinfectant. Environ-mentally-safe cleaning products are also readily available from your local health shop.**

- **Throw out artificial air fresheners, as some emit toxic odours that can cause cancer. Many contain lethal substances such as ethanol, formaldehyde, phenol and xylene. Instead, use proper ventilation, fresh flowers or aromatherapy essential oils on a pot pourri.**
- **When using scented candles, make sure that they are made from plant- or bees-wax which contain pure essential oils and not synthetic fragrances.**
- **If you are redecorating, try to use natural furnishings that have not been treated by chemicals.**
- **Avoid exposure to all products that contains methylene chloride and benzene. These are found in paint strippers and aerosol spray paint, and have been linked to cancer in both humans and animals.**
- **When using facial and body creams, choose natural, environmentally friendly products.**
- **Cut down or eliminate the use of perfumes and colognes: many are made from petrochemicals and synthetic toxic materials which can compromise your immune system. Use natural essential oils instead.**
- **Studies have shown that as many as 20% of non-Hodgkin's lymphoma are related to the use of artificial hair colouring. Use a non-toxic, plant based, biodegradable hair-colourant instead.**
- **Use a fluoride-free toothpaste (there is a debate as the moment as to how safe it is).**
- **Avoid using commercial deodorants and antiperspirants. These products frequently contain harmful ingredients such as aluminium which has been linked with Alzheimer's disease.**
- **Bring plants into your home as they combat air pollution. Remember to remove them from your bedroom at night, when plants generally absorb oxygen and give off carbon dioxide.**
- **Wear clothing made of natural fibres, ie cotton and linen. When washing your clothes, use an environmentally safe washing powder such as Ecovert. And finally, if you need to dry-clean your clothes, always make sure you air them well before putting them back in your wardrobe.**

POOR NUTRITION

Nutrition has a critical role to play in maintaining our body's health. A poor diet can and does have a negative effect on our well-being, so it's crucial to watch not just what but also how you eat. Here are some of the ways that poor nutrition can influence your health:

Dehydration: The body's cells contain up to 75% water, and need water to function efficiently. Dehydration is a factor present in many of the clients I see. You should drink 8 – 10 glasses of water every day to hydrate your body properly.

Food Allergies: Intolerances or allergies to foods occur as a result of the body not being able to process or assimilate food properly. Many allergies are caused by foods eaten on a regular basis: this includes wheat and dairy products. The body likes a variety of food to help it maximise energy. If an intolerance occurs, ailments like chest infections, skin disorders or migraines may result. So vary your intake of foods.

"Unnatural" foods: avoid processed foods and food that has been treated with pesticides or radiation, and try to ensure that as much as possible of what you eat is whole, pure, natural and fresh. Choose organic or home-grown foods. Food should not need added pesticides, extra salt or sugar. The spices, sauces and condiments that people use are sometimes irritating to the body, and should be used sparingly. Foods high in white sugar should be avoided entirely. Other things to avoid – or to be taken in moderation - include fried foods, foods high in fats, white rice, pasteurised milk products, and white flour which is high in gluten (which can cause celiac disease).

Over-acidic body systems: When the body is acidic, it becomes ill. Our intake of alkaline foods should be 80% to 20% acidic. 6 vegetables and 2 fruits could make up the alkaline portion we need, whilst one protein and one starch could provide the 20% acidic. Meats contain uric acid and should be eaten sparingly. Uric acid can cause high blood pressure, gout, arthritis, urinary tract disorders and other problems. Building up an excess of acid in our bodies is not wise, as it can create a lot of health ailments. So eat more vegetables and fruit, more fish, and less meat, especially red meat.

Don't over-eat: When the body is overweight, the heart has to pump harder, blood circulation is slower, and more pressure is placed on the feet and legs. Sometimes the colon will prolapse from the extra weight, which in turn puts pressure on the other organs. A person will have less energy when over-weight, and often their self-esteem is lowered. Food should never control us – as the old saying goes, you should eat to live, not live to eat! We should only consume the foods that will meet our need to have a chemically balanced, healthy body. It is also important to thoroughly masticate your food, ie to chew for at least 30 seconds on each mouthful.

Watch the way you cook: Steamed or raw vegetables are better for you than boiled vegetables. Similarly, grilled foods are better than shallow- or deep-fried foods. If you are shallow-frying foods, use an unsaturated oil. Finally, microwave ovens can also destroy some of the useful enzymes in food, and should be avoided.

So in conclusion, the essence of good nutrition is to eat natural, pure, whole and fresh foods as often as possible. Do so, and watch your health ailments disappear!

FEARS

A fear is defined as an emotion caused by an impending danger or pain, making us afraid or anxious. Fears take many different forms, and they can have a huge impact on our lives, stopping us from moving forward. Some people are afraid of animals or insects: dogs, spiders, mice, rats and snakes (I don't like snakes!). Other fears concern certain situations: agoraphobia (fear of open spaces), or fear of crowds, public speaking, flying, water and so on. Finally, there are more deep-seated fears: fear of death, failure, authority, rejection, loneliness, poverty, losing control and so on. The list of fears is endless!

Some fears are stored in the unconscious mind and are embedded so deeply that the conscious mind is not aware of them. These fears may come out in dreams. As an example, in my clinic I saw a young child who had sleeping problems and nightmares. Her fears stemmed from an unpleasant experience whilst in hospital. The first stage in overcoming fears is to recognise them, and to work out where they might have come from. In this case, I gave the child homeopathic remedies to help overcome her fear and happily she moved on.

So how can fears affect your health? They can lead to palpitations, tightness in the chest, freezing on the spot, or as in the case above, sleeplessness. They can also be the root cause of conditions such as panic / anxiety attacks, cystitis and headaches. Unconscious fears often have a more subtle effect, where a feeling of unease leads to negativity, low self esteem and ultimately a depleted immune system, which in turn results in a tendency for such people to catch every bug going. It is my experience and strong belief that positive people are the healthiest people!

Many fears and phobias result from a shocking experience in the past, or from a slow erosion of the person's confidence. I myself have a great fear of failure and of authority, which I can now see stems back to my schooldays. Some of the teachers I had made me believe that I was lazy with certain subjects, leading me to lose belief in myself and my abilities. But by recognising and acknowledging my fears, I have learned to accept and overcome them, and not let them take over my life.

If you feel that you have fears that are taking over your life, try the following steps to help overcome them:

- **Share your feelings of fear with other people. It is important to be honest with your feelings, rather than trying to deny them or pretend that they do not exist**
- **Face your fear and don't let it hold you back. You will feel so much better, and even if you fail, keep trying (although I still don't like them, I faced my fear of snakes by holding one at a children's reptile party recently!)**
- **Learn to trust others in order to feel safe in the world.**

Remember the saying: "Fear knocked on the door, love answered, nobody was there."

ANGER

Have you ever seen a person mad with anger? Eyes bulging, face red, fists clenched, head looking like it's about to explode? When someone is this angry, it's actually quite easy to see the effect it's having on their body: high blood pressure, fast but shallow breathing, rapid heart-beat and palpitations, constricted muscles: all things that can and do have a negative impact on our health. In many ways, anger is the opposite of love. Violent anger is often a symptom of pent-up rage, erupting in destructive ways, and it can also be a sign that you need professional help.

Anger is a destructive emotion, not just of physical things, but also of inner peace, harmony and balance. Some people are afraid to express their anger because they feel too vulnerable. In this instance, anger can go inwards, causing more imbalance in the body. Suppressed anger can be just as destructive as expressed anger.

From a homeopathic perspective, anger can be stored in the liver, heart and lungs. In other words, if you are angry all the time, this can have a direct impact on the energy and the proper functioning of these organs. The liver is the second largest organ in the body (after the skin), and it plays an essential role in removing toxins from the body. Excess anger can put extra pressure on the liver, leading to poor detoxing, and hence to fatigue, especially on rising in the morning, and to conditions like irritable bowel syndrome and skin disorders. Excess anger in the heart and the lungs can lead to feelings of sadness and disappointment, resulting in depression, respiratory problems and heart problems.

Angry people will often suffer from over-stimulation of the nervous system, and this in turn can result in conditions such as migraines, high blood pressure, arthritis, psoriasis and so on. In my experience, it's clear that there is a link between anger and certain ailments. So what can be done to dissolve feelings of anger in the body, and to help the angry person to put their body back into balance?

The first thing an angry person should do is forgive him/herself, and let go of old hurts, past injustices and great disappointments. The next thing to do is to "forgive thy enemy": this is therapeutic to the person forgiving (ie the angry person). Forgiveness changes negative thoughts, energy and cells to positive ones, and thus lowers the blood pressure, releases the tension held in the joints (ie arthritis) and helps to balance the energy around the heart.

It also helps to let your anger out. Find a method that suits you (and that doesn't scare those around you!) – punch a pillow, go for a run, or scream at the top of your voice in your car. I find homeopathic medicines such as Nux Vomica, Lycopodium and Nat Mur can help people to express their anger, not in violent outbursts, but by gently releasing pent-up emotions and allowing them to verbalise their feelings more appropriately. All these remedies can help people to feel more confident and have less need to prove themselves.

Finally, I also find that affirmations are very useful in helping to release anger from the body. Repeat the following phrases to yourself daily, three times in the morning and the evening:

"I love myself easily from head to toe. I send love to all my enemies."

When we feel anger, we resist the joy of life and the magnificence of our being.

LOSS & SADNESS

Nobody goes through life without experiencing a loss, be it the loss of a loved one, a pet, a job, one's childhood, or children leaving home to go to college. Mourning and coming to terms with a loss are a natural part of life, and are things that we must all go though at some stage our lives. But if we let the sense of loss and sadness overtake our lives, it can have a detrimental effect on our health. Sadness and a sense of loss can harm the body in many ways, leading to conditions such as depression, insomnia, migraines, irritable bowel syndrome, arthritis, hypertension, fatigue and so on – the list is endless. In extreme cases, people can literally die from the sadness of a broken heart: I know of a number of cases where a wife had passed away one day and the husband has followed within a few days.

The loss may be felt as an abandonment, making you feel shocked, wounded or betrayed. You may no longer feel connected to the world, making you isolate yourself and leading to feelings of loneliness. The sadness may be felt especially in the heart and lungs. You may become very angry, either with yourself or with anyone connected to the sense of loss. If the anger is not acknowledged, it can go inwards and result in depression. You may also feel guilt, which eats away at your insides, leading to early morning waking, unwanted thoughts, fatigue, palpitations or "butterflies" in your tummy.

When a loss occurs, people sometimes put armour around their heart. At first this may seem protective, but in reality it can stop you from feeling pain, sadness or indeed any joy in your life. So what can be done to overcome the sense of grief and loss we may be feeling?

When we lose a loved one, we feel we are never going to meet them again, we feel they are gone forever. But we should remember that we are a "spirit with a body" and not a "body with a spirit." The spirit never dies! We are all on earth going to school to learn our life lessons. One of those life lessons is to experience a loss so we can try and understand mortality and what lies beyond life.

It is OK to feel grief and sadness, but ultimately each of us needs to come to terms with our loss. That means resolving to live life more fully in each and every moment, rather than hanging on to the incomplete past or shielding ourselves from the present. As much as we would like to be in control of our life and situations, we really have to trust in the natural flow of events. Whether we like it or not, life is given to us to live in the moment, since it can be taken away from us in the blink of an eye. So to help overcome grief and sadness, you need to work on changing your sad cells to happy ones. Live in the moment – not in the past or in the future – and any time you feel yourself becoming overwhelmed with sadness, say these words to yourself to help you become happier:

"I breathe in love and light to all the cells in my body. I live in the now. I trust in the flow of life."

The homeopathic remedies Nat Mur and Aconite can also be used to treat loss and sadness. Nat Mur heals the pain by helping people to connect to the joy in their lives, rather than to the sadness. Aconite helps people to get over the shock often associated with a loss, and hence makes them feel more relaxed in themselves.

GUILT & SHAME

Guilt can take away all the joy from your life. You may find yourself saying "I should be doing this, I should be doing that" instead of "I am doing this, I am doing that." No matter what you do or however much you succeed, if you live in the world of "I should", you will never feel you have accomplished anything, and will continue always to want to achieve more. This sense of non-achievement may concern your relationship with yourself or others, your job, your housework, your education and so on.

You may have internalised the moral code of your family or society, or you may have developed your own code through the course of your life experiences. Sometimes you may be internalising the guilt of others which needs to be put back where it belongs.

In some ways guilt can contribute to your maturity through a sense of taking responsibility for your life. As you mature, it can serve to remind you of your responsibilities towards other people and to refine your evolving sense of integrity.

So much for the positive aspects of guilt: in its negative aspect, guilt is often connected with a complete perfectionist attitude towards yourself and others, in which you are not allowed to make mistakes. Guilt can also stay lodged in your psyche, eroding your sense of self-worth. It can produce low self-esteem and make the sufferer feel unworthy. It may erupt into a crisis of confidence where you begin to doubt your own abilities. Guilt is an internalisation of shame, where you feel you have not lived up to your standards or code of honour.

The first step in healing guilt and shame is to share your imperfection. Be honest about your mistakes and shortcomings, rather than denying them or pretending they do not exist. It is usually shame that makes us try to cover things up. But it is better to expose whatever you feel guilty about, because it then loses some of its power over you. Letting go of the resistance frees you. In letting go, you are learning to open up and trust others again.

I have seen several cases in my clinics where a person's guilty feelings have led directly to a depleted immune system, which in turn has led to the person becoming repeatedly ill. Often, the guilt has also been directly responsible for high cholesterol levels. These people tend to be very loyal and duty-bound, striving for perfection and dwelling on their perceived failures as opposed to what they have achieved. The "cure" for such people is to acknowledge their guilt, then to use affirmations and homeopathic remedies (for example Aurum or Arsenicum) to boost their self-esteem, which in turn makes them happier in themselves. As I have mentioned elsewhere, happy people tend to be healthy people (and vice versa!).

The radical psychiatrist R D Laing argued that true guilt is the product of not fulfilling your obligation to yourself to realise your true potential and be yourself. Healing guilt involves taking the risk of reconnecting with your deeper sense of self.

So to help overcome guilt and shame, follow these wise words: "Be yourself at all times and speak the truth powerfully and lovingly." When guilt is out of your life, you have less need to be serious and so see the wealth of humour that runs through life: thus joy returns and you feel happier and healthier.

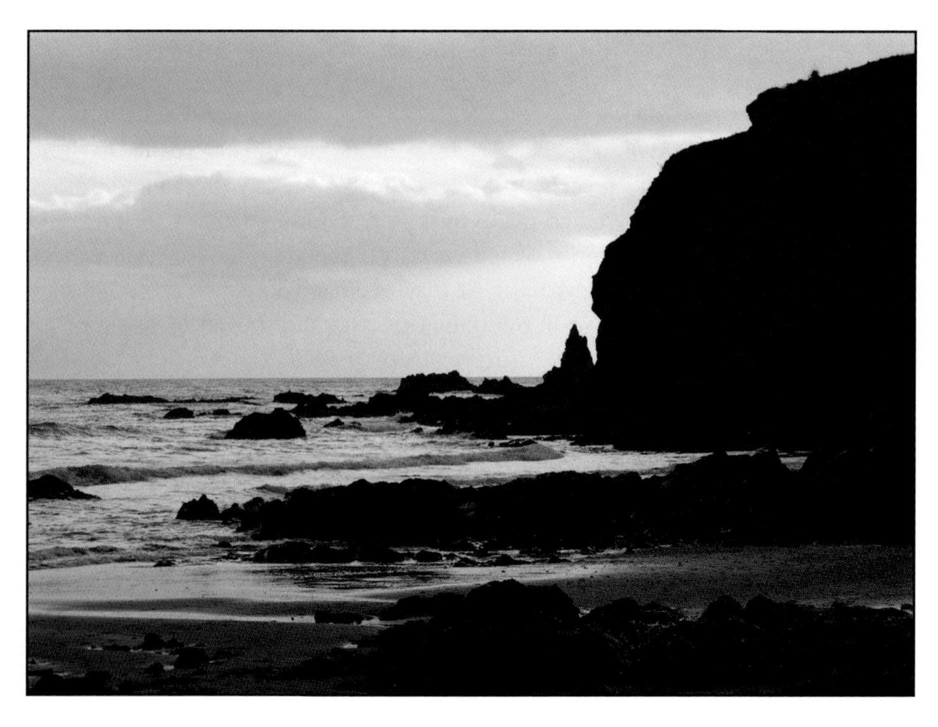

"Forgiveness is the key to happiness. Forgive yourself first and then your enemies."

CONSTITUTIONAL & GENETIC WEAKNESS

Have you ever wondered why some people can smoke for years and never get lung cancer, whilst other people can get it from secondary smoking? Or why is it that certain conditions like asthma or eczema seem to run in families? Or that some work colleagues seem to pick up every 'flu bug going, whereas other lucky ones never seem to get the sniffles! And why, on our honeymoon in India, did I suffer from several tummy bugs, whilst my husband sailed through without a problem?!

The answer to these questions often lies in constitutional or genetic weaknesses. Your constitution reflects your genetic make-up. It is the sum of your inborn physical and emotional characteristics – the general condition and character of your body.

To help me identify imbalances in people's bodies, I use a combination of muscle-testing and iridology. With iridology, I look into the irises, and using a lens and torch, I can gather information on people's constitutional strengths and weaknesses. One look at the eye reveals what type of constitution you have: perhaps you have a tendency towards a nervous disposition, or are more susceptible to rheumatic or arthritic conditions, or are prone to allergies.

Our individual genetic dispositions and hereditary tendencies are directly related to the strengths and weaknesses we are born with, and often determine the type of conditions to which we are more prone. Some people have weak or sensitive digestive systems, some are born with strong lung tissue, some have weak livers, and some have strong kidneys: to some extent it is a lottery!

We all have inherent strengths and weaknesses that we carry through life, although this is not to say that we will necessarily suffer from certain ailments: just an increased likelihood.

Our lifestyle habits, our environment and our stress levels all affect our health and well-being. For instance, emotional stress affects each and every one of us, but in different ways: in one person it might lead to stomach ulcers, for another a migraine, and for someone else a skin complaint.

Through knowledge of an individual's constitution, we can thus discover not only those types of symptoms to which he or she might be susceptible, but also the causes of the symptoms – for example if the constitution indicates that the person is susceptible to hyperacidity and related conditions (like stomach ulcers, rheumatism, arthritis and minor skin complaints), then he or she should avoid, or keep to an absolute minimum, the high acid-forming foods such as white bread, red meat, citrus fruits, wheat products, coffee, tea, alcohol etc. Acid forming foods like these will only serve to irritate the underlying tendency.

The human body is an incredible creation, very strong and resilient. Symptoms only follow if after a period of time, we cause them through our constitutional type, our lifestyle, diet, psychological stress, lack of proper exercise, environmental toxins, climate etc. If we choose to pursue a manner of lifestyle that puts stress on our inherent weaknesses, sooner or later symptoms will manifest themselves. Unless we take remedial measures to deal with the root causes of the conditions, then clinical "disease" may set in.

3
GENERAL HEALTH

ANTIBIOTICS

Q: *As you are complementary health practitioner, please could you give me your views on antibiotics? There seems to have been a lot of bad press about them recently – a lot of it amazingly from conventional doctors!*

A: Antibiotics are one of the most commonly prescribed drugs. If you go along to your doctor with something like a sore throat, there is a good chance he will prescribe antibiotics to make you better. However, many health professionals, including conventional doctors, now believe that antibiotics have been prescribed too readily. There are several problems with the over-prescription of antibiotics:

- **every time you take an antibiotic, you risk weakening your body's own natural healing mechanism, and killing off friendly bacteria that aid digestion and enhance your immunity.**
- **antibiotics can be prescribed incorrectly, eg antibiotics only work on bacterial infections, and have no effect on viral, fungal or parasitic infections**
- **if you take too many antibiotics, you may develop a resistance to them, making them ineffective should you develop a very serious condition such as meningitis, or increasing your risk of contracting MRSA.**

I am not suggesting for one moment that antibiotics should not be used: but rather that they should not be used willy nilly, as sometimes seems to be the case nowadays. If a stressed office worker has a recurring sore throat, and four bouts of antibiotics have failed to shift it, clearly the suggested cure is not working, and a different approach needs to be tried!

Some homeopathic remedies work like antibiotics. But the biggest difference is that the homeopath will look at the causes of the illness as well as the symptoms. In the case of our office worker, it may be that he gets a sore throat every time he gets stressed at work: so the homeopath would look at ways of coping better with that stress, rather than just giving something to cure the sore throat.

I have four children aged between 8 and 13, and not one of them has ever had an antibiotic. Trust me, they have had the usual childhood suspects of sore throats, chest infections and ear infections, but I have successfully used homeopathic remedies to boost their immune system and help them to override the infections themselves. It works for adults too: my husband and I have never had an antibiotic in 17 years since I began studying homeopathy. The majority of people I see in my clinics ask for help in boosting their immune system, which in many cases has been depleted by the overuse of antibiotics and other suppressive medicines. If you are in any doubt as to the seriousness of an infection, then of course you should consult with your GP ... but you - and indeed your GP! - should also be aware that there are effective, natural alternatives to antibiotics, such as homeopathic remedies, pre- or pro-biotics, and natural, live yogurt: ask a registered health professional for more information.

BOOSTING YOUR IMMUNE SYSTEM

Q: *Can you give me any tips on keeping my family's immune systems strong through the cold winter months? We all seem to be suffering from repeated coughs and colds at the moment.*

A: I'm sorry to hear you and your family are having a rough time with all the coughs and colds! Of course, a weak immune system can lead to frequent colds and infections. A strong immune system, on the other hand, gives you a greater resistance not just to colds and infections, but also to auto-immune diseases such as cancer and arthritis (an auto-immune disease is one where the body's defences attack its own cells).

Your immune system becomes more sluggish in cold weather, and can also be severely weakened by a number of factors: these include excess alcohol, cigarettes, a high-fat or protein-deficient diet, lack of sleep, or stress. As well as avoiding these factors, try the following tips to help maintain your positive health and well-being:

1. Eat a mucus-free diet

A number of foods create too much mucus in the diet, especially milk and dairy products, eggs and red meat (some people are particularly susceptible to this). Excess mucus clogs up the lymphatic system, so try to cut down on or avoid these foods. Try soya or rice milk, make your own nutritious, organic soups, and eat plenty of steamed vegetables with your chicken or fish.

2. Keep drinking water

When you are under viral attack, your immune system needs to get rid of toxic debris, which it does via the kidneys and bladder. This is why frequent trips to the loo are often a sign of infection. Drink tepid water, herbal teas, diluted fruit juices or vegetable juices to help the kidneys to do their job. Cut back on coffee, tea and alcohol, and drink at least 8 - 10 glasses of water daily.

3. Take Vitamin C

Countless studies have shown that Vitamin C helps to fight off colds. Add the juice of half a lemon to a mug of boiling water, and have this as your hot drink in the morning (you can add a teaspoon of manuka honey to make it sweeter). Or eat 2 room temperature kiwi fruits daily, preferably before your meals (kiwis enhance the digestive enzymes in the stomach and aid digestion).

4. Maintain adequate temperature and humidity levels

Central heating can dry up your mucous membranes, so humidify your room with a saucer of water near the heater to moisten the air and help prevent sinusitis.

5. Exercise

Make sure you continue to exercise during the winter months even if only for a short period during your lunch-break. The pineal gland in your brain craves as much light as possible to alleviate the effects of SAD (seasonal affective disorder) and to make your cells happier: so make sure you get outside when it's light, and don't stay indoors in an office all day.

6. Stay positive and happy

Think positively. Say the following affirmation three times in the morning and three times in the evening:

"I crave only healthy foods and beverages, my immune system is strong and everything is in divine and perfect order right now."

This affirmation will help you to stop eating comforting junk food when you are feeling sorry for yourself. Introduce nuts and seeds into your diet instead – they are a much healthier option to feed your brain cells.

If all this fails to help, then go and see your local natural health practitioner, and try homeopathic medicine to boost your immune system.

BOOSTING YOUR SELF ESTEEM

Our self-esteem is very much linked to feelings of connection with – and acceptance by – other people. When we feel isolated and alienated, our sense of self is undermined and we may suffer from a sense of worthlessness. Lack of self-esteem can be produced by undermining experiences in childhood, when we are perhaps made to feel that love and approval are conditional upon us fulfilling the expectations of others. Too much criticism can weaken our sense of self when we are growing up.

Low self-esteem is endemic in a society that pays lip service to the importance of the individual and his or her unique needs. That same society is mainly concerned with educating each of us to be a cog in the wheel, rather than encouraging us to discover our own true destiny.

When we do not feel confident, we retreat into a shell, not daring to risk rejection. We do not have the confidence to risk exposure to anything, so we may keep many aspects of ourselves hidden.

The homeopathic remedies described below can help people who are stuck in their energy pattern. The remedies help you to let go of a negative self-image by gaining a greater self awareness of your value in life. We each must learn to accept and to love ourselves fully. Try extending to yourself the compassion you can feel for other people who are struggling.

AMBRA GRISEA: Person is extremely shy and comes out with foolish comments when embarrassed.

CAL CARB: Person worries about their mental abilities and dreads being exposed as a "fraud." This remedy is healing for people who are slow at grasping things.

LYCOPODIUM: Person worries too much about the future, their security, and has a great fear about losing control of their lives. They may also crave sweet things.

SILICEA: Person feels shy and awkward in social situations. A lack of confidence in their work abilities makes them overly conscientious about details.

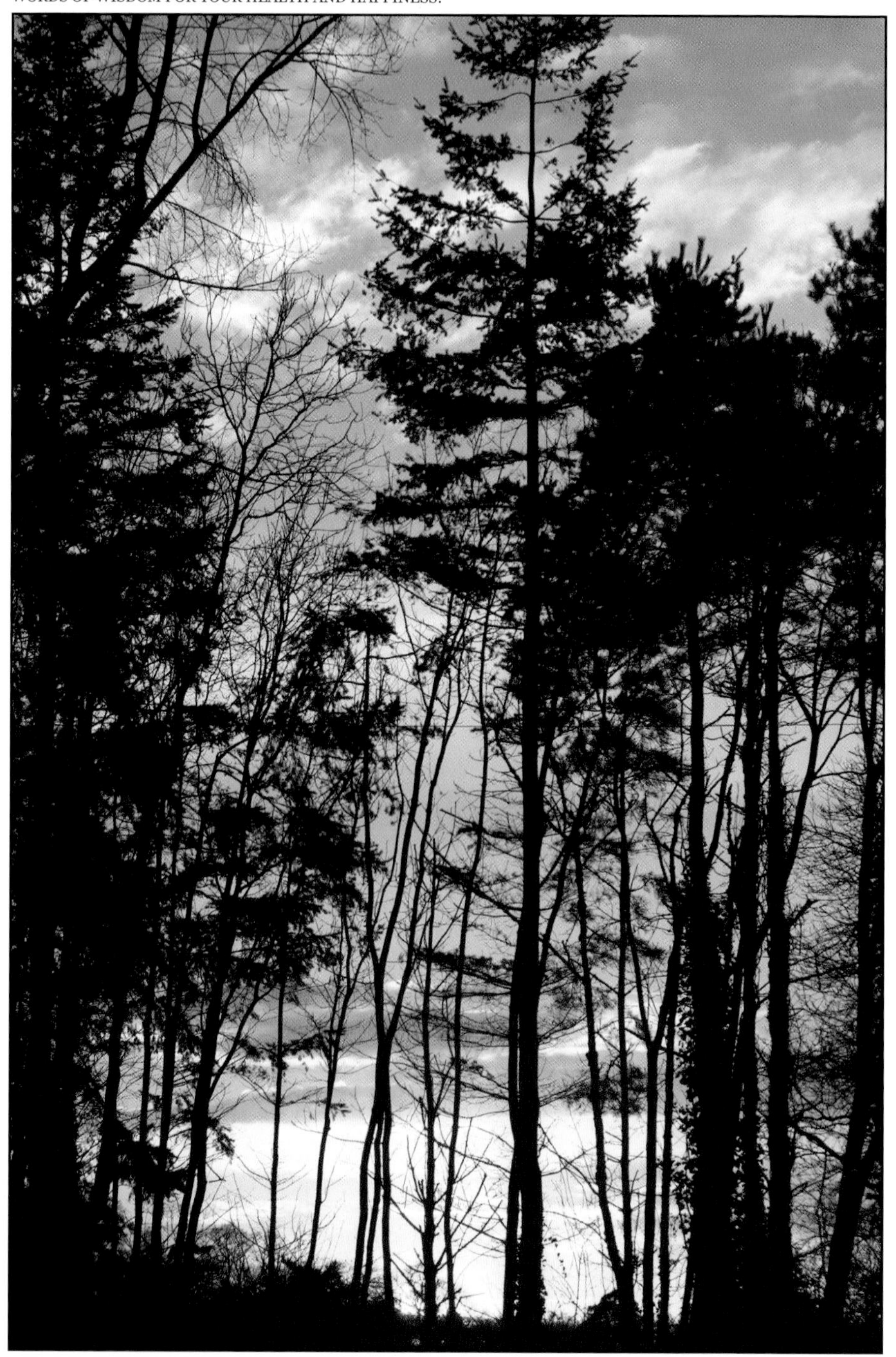

"In order to change the world, first change yourself." ~ Shaun de Warren

DIAGNOSTIC MUSCLE TESTING / KINESIOLOGY

One of the diagnostic techniques I employ in my clinics is kinesiology, also known as muscle testing. I use it in a variety of ways: to help pinpoint the maintaining cause of disease, to find any emotional blockages, to identify allergies, and to prescribe the best homeopathic remedies to help boost the immune system and balance the body's energy. It is a relatively simple technique but is amazingly powerful and accurate.

I find muscle testing incredibly useful in locating some of the more unusual causes of imbalance in the body – for example, metal allergies, electromagnetic stress or geopathic stress. It's also very good at determining the exact cause of illness. I once saw a child who had been given six lots of antibiotics for a sore throat, but who was still suffering from the condition. I used kinesiology to diagnose that the problem was viral, and not bacterial. Antibiotics only work on bacterial infections, so no wonder the poor child was not getting any better! I gave her homeopathic remedies to boost her immune system and to help her body overcome the viral infection, and am delighted to report that she made a full recovery. This is a perfect example of the powerful nature and effectiveness of muscle testing.

Kinesiology is defined as the study of muscles and their movement, as applied to physical conditions in the body. It originated in 1964 through the scientific work of American Dr George J Goodheart. In the 1970's, Dr John Diamond refined the technique into a new discipline which he called behavioural kinesiology. He discovered that indicator muscles would become stronger or weaker in the presence of positive or negative emotional and intellectual stimuli. So, for example, a smile will make you test strong, but thinking something negative like "I hate you!" will make you test weak.

I first discovered muscle testing in 1990, when I was studying nutrition and testing for food allergies. Later, when one of my daughters was ill with a high fever, I found it was brilliant to help me choose the right remedies to bring down her fever and speed her recovery. I then worked closely with a leading UK health practitioner, Roger Dyson, who taught me his diagnostic muscle testing technique, which focuses on discovering why the body goes out of balance.

From my own findings, I believe that the body has an innate memory or intelligence that is in many respects far superior to the mind. The mind may choose to forget a sad or painful event, but the body stores the memory. If the cells are not released of this emotional block, then physical ailments can develop, leading to disease. Of course, everyone has a different story, a different block and a different, unique remedy requirement to help heal themselves.

In my workshops, I always use muscle testing to demonstrate to people the power of positive and negative thought patterns. Negative thoughts can detrimental to our health, whilst positive thoughts strengthen the body and help us to be happier and more joyful in ourselves.

EXERCISE: SHIFTING BRAIN CHEMISTRY & BEHAVIOUR NATURALLY!

What if the world of science discovered a pill that could instantly alleviate depression and anxiety, and also help a person to lose weight, live longer and feel happier? And what if this pill was freely available to everybody without a doctor's prescription, and available at a relatively low price – or even for free? Wouldn't everyone clamour to buy the pill?

Well, such a "cure-all" does exist, and its effectiveness is backed up by countless scientific studies: and it is called EXERCISE!

Studies show that aerobic exercise in particular – running, jogging, stair-climbing, swimming, cycling and brisk walking – increases the production of the brain chemical serotonin and other feel-good neurotransmitters.

Since suffering depression some in my 20's, I introduced exercise into my life plan, and have never looked back since. Anti-depressants helped temporarily, but were not the answer. I am realistic: I know most people consider exercise to be boring, painful and time-consuming. I often feel the same way! But in my clinics, I regularly prescribe exercise as well as homeopathic medicines.

I sometimes find jogging boring, especially the first 15 minutes, as the feet and body feel heavy and unresponsive. But somewhere thereafter, the rhythm sets in, and I feel my breath deepen so that my lungs can take in more air. And after my run around the local GAA ground (often with 4 kids and 2 dogs in tow!), I feel exuberant and yet relaxed. Any worries or cares I had before the run seem insignificant afterwards.

Many studies also show that exercise increases the quality of a person's sleep and reduces insomnia. There are many forms of exercise to suit each individual and lifestyle, be it jogging, brisk walking, trampolining, hip-hoping to your local dance class, salsa, yoga, tai chi, or any of the organised sports like hurling, soccer and so on.

Yoga helps one to meditate and lose negative thought patterns. It is especially useful for people who complain that they have difficulty meditating because their mind is too busy or noisy, or who fall asleep during meditation.

So as the end of the summer approaches, go on! – make yourself a promise to introduce exercise into your life and feel the uplifting effects of serotonin. It uplifts you naturally, alleviates fatigue, and makes the sad cells in our body happy. Surely all traditional and complementary health practitioners should be pushing more exercise on our prescription pads instead of medication?

FIGHTING THE FLABBY TUMMY!

I was in a local health store recently and got talking to a couple of ladies there. They asked me if there was anything I could suggest for "unwanted flabby tummy" which they still had despite losing weight. This problem seems to be very prevalent, mainly among the female of the species! In my clinics I have found there to be two main reasons for this condition: candida and hormone imbalance.

Candida is an overgrowth of yeast in the body fed by too much sugar. This overgrowth causes bloatedness and hinders the digestive process. Solutions are as follows:

- **Cut out sugar and sugary foods from your diet**
- **Cut out foods which contain yeast, ie cakes, biscuits, processed white and brown bread – instead opt for soda, rye or spelt breads (these are also much higher in fibre)**
- **Try to avoid antibiotics, and use natural medicines to boost the immune system. Antibiotics can kill off friendly bacteria and cause candida.**

For more, see the separate article on candida.

It's hard to believe that hormones can create a bloated tummy, but it's true. There are two homeopathic remedies that can help, depending on your symptoms. Choose the one that most closely matches your situation. If you think both remedies describe you, take both. Take a 30 potency am and pm for two weeks, then take a break for two weeks and watch the changes occur. You may need to repeat the prescription of homeopathic medicine as the blood cells change every 120 days, so repeat monthly for no more than 3 months (two weeks on, two weeks off).

SEPIA is a common housewives' remedy, where the woman feels as if she never gets a break from the grind of housework, kids, chores etc and never has time for herself. Symptoms include a flabby midline of tummy, and feeling bloated. It may feel like your bladder is weak, especially if you sneeze or cough. You may also feel irritable and indifferent to loved ones on occasions, crave chocolate and have a low sex drive.

PULSATILLA helps to balance the hormones and clean out the lymphatic system (the drainage system in the body). To improve things, try cutting out cheese and dairy products that can clog up the system and trust that your body gets enough calcium from your dark green veg. People in a "Pulsatilla state" say "poor me", they feel unloved and unappreciated, and feel like they are always taking responsibility for doing everything. This makes them very needy, and they become the nagging housewife, blaming their loved ones all the time. They smile outwardly but seethe inwardly. This builds up resentment that can ultimately affect their hormones, and hence lead to symptoms like PMT, breast tenderness, period problems, and feeling low prior to periods. They crave stodgy foods, cigarettes or alcohol to make them feel better, but of course long term these are of no help.

IRIDOLOGY

Iridology is the study of the iris, the coloured part of the eye. It is a non-invasive therapy that allows the practitioner, using a torch and lens, to determine information on the patient's health and well-being.

Iridology was founded in 1866 by Dr Ignatz van Peczely of Budapest, Hungary. He discovered nature's records in the eye quite by accident. As a ten year old boy, he nursed an owl with a broken leg back to health. As the owl recovered, he noticed that a marking in a part of its eye changed. This ultimately led him to map the whole human eye, with each part of the iris corresponding to a different part of the body. The link is the optical nerve. Via the optical nerve, the iris is connected into the central nervous system and hence to every other part of the body. Markings, colorations and features in the iris can thus indicate problem areas in the body, imbalances, constitutional weaknesses and so on.

The outer zone of the iris represents the skin, moving inwards is the lymphatic system, and then towards the centre of the iris come various organs. To the iridologist, the iris is like a clock face, with each area representing a part of the body: for example, the brain area is represented between 11 and 1 o'clock, whilst the stomach area is seen closest to the pupil. Some organs are represented in just one eye (such as the liver on the right iris), whilst others, like the heart, are seen on the both irises. Iridologists do not typically name diseases: rather they only see inflammation, weaknesses or toxic build-up in the body.

Enough science! I thought it would be more interesting to give a practical example of iridology in action:

A client presents with indigestion and heartburn. Using a high powered torch and lens, I would look into the stomach and colon areas in the iris. A plugged, toxic or ineffective digestive system is very easily seen in the iris. If the area is white in colour, this tells me that the person is producing too much acid. A grey to dark grey colour indicates low or no acid, and poor digestion of proteins. By using iridology to diagnose the cause of the condition, I can then give the patient the appropriate homeopathic remedies and dietary advice to help them improve their health.

Iridology can give information not only on your current state of your health, but also on inherited weaknesses. If the eyes reveal an inherited weakness in the lymphatic system (the drainage system in our bodies), then necessary precautions can be taken in diet and lifestyle to help stay healthy - otherwise repeated colds, breast lumps and cysts can occur.

If you would like to learn more about iridology, I recommend "Immunology & Iridology" by John Andrews (see www.johnandrewsiridology.net).

STAYING HEALTHY WITH THE SEASONS

As the end of summer approaches and autumn comes into our horizons, some parents may be sighing with relief as their loved ones return to school ("Phew! – Some time to myself at last!").

This seasonal change marks the shift from the outward expression of spring and summer to the inward focus of autumn and winter. Some people are very sensitive to this change (myself included), so how can we ensure we stay healthy through the autumnal and winter months?

Remember that late summer is the beginning of the harvest time. Ripe fruits are falling to the ground, and vegetables are growing plump and fat all around. Weather permitting, we may eat as lightly as feels good, but as we move towards the autumn equinox, the cycle of darkness becomes dominant and our balance shifts inward. This is a time when you can begin your building and toning program, which includes diet and exercise.

A building diet will give you a greater proportion of protein-rich foods, whole grains, seeds, nuts and beans. But remember that your diet should always contain a good percentage of fresh fruit and vegetables too for a proper alkaline balance. We naturally want to eat heavier type protein in the winter months. I would also recommend a few days monthly (before it gets too cold) to do a juice cleanse to help eliminate the toxins from the richer type foods.

Keep sugar to a minimum (I strongly believe that the high consumption of sugars in our diet - from cereals, soft drinks, alcohol, salad dressings, cakes etc – contributes to major health problems in people today). The physical highs and lows caused by sugar, and the resulting mental imbalance - which includes depression, anxiety and irritability - may indeed have created the need for the first mental institute in the 17th century. Remember that the brain cells are most sensitive to changes in blood sugar levels.

The following suggestions can be of help during the autumn and winter months:

- **Keep exercise going as long as possible with outdoor activities and sports (yes, I am still jogging around the local GAA ground!), or join a**

gym or local exercise classes

- **Eat slowly, chew your food well, and DON'T OVERLOAD!**
- **Proteins - ie meats, eggs and starches - should be taken in moderation and only in proportion to the work one does**
- **Food combining (separating proteins and starches based on the Hay diet) helps to keep your weight under control and your digestion to work more efficiently**
- **Taken before mealtimes, two teaspoons of organic cider apple vinegar enhances digestion**
- **Get out in the daylight during the winter months, even if it's a cloudy day. The pineal gland in the brain loves the sunlight and this enhances the feel-good factor.**

As the seasonal transition takes place, your diet, exercise regime and lifestyle affect all aspects of your life: your work, productivity, personality, sleep patterns and dreams, how you feel from day to day, your good or poor health and well-being, and where you live in your mind. So let's be positive and move with the flow – that's the real way to grow, so let's go!

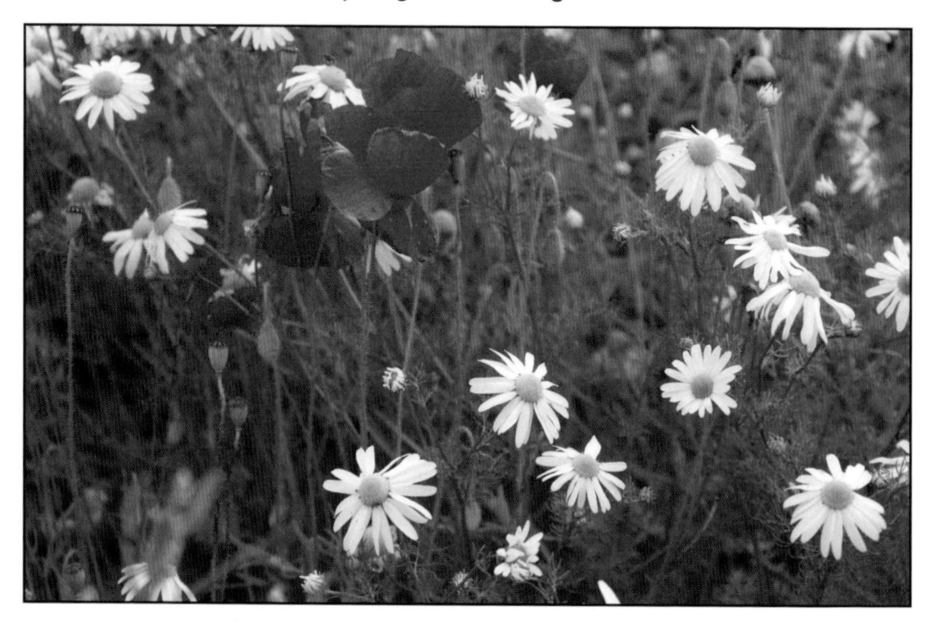

"The mind is a garden that occasionally needs weeding."

THE BODY REMEMBERS

When we are totally happy and relaxed, the energy in each cell in our body is good and we enjoy good health. But the reverse is also true: anxiety, fear, anger, hurt, criticism, jealousy, negative thoughts, losses and shocks held in the body can and do affect the physical body, sometimes resulting in illness. We feel upset in the morning, and come out in a rash that afternoon. We feel unspeakably angry with someone at work one day, and the next day we lose our voice. If we find it difficult to express grief, we may develop depression, asthma or the unshed tears of chronic catarrh or sinus problems. More deeply suppressed emotions frequently take six months to crystallise into illness. Often cancer develops two years after a trauma or the death of someone we love.

The body remembers but the head denies it. If I were to prescribe homeopathic medicine based on what is being said to me alone, I am sure that the client would not get the good results necessary for them to move on! In other words we need to be living less in our heads and more in our bodies. We need to understand that ailments come up to talk to us in order to let us know that our body needs balancing. To get the best results in healing, all aspects of a person need to be addressed – not just the physical aspect in isolation, but also our mental, emotional and spiritual sides. I strongly believe that this holistic approach is the only way forward!

As soon as we open up and release the tensions in the body with love, forgiveness, compassion, awareness and understanding, then divine energy flows and we can be healed.

Some people do not find it easy in their hearts to forgive and move on. I use homeopathic medicines to help to remove such blockages, to get the body's energy flowing again, and to help people to be more aware and to release the anger that is eating away at their cells.

Our cells are constantly dying and being replaced. In seven years, every cell in our bodies has been renewed, so we have the possibility of totally transforming our body, at least within seven years. One of the reasons we do not heal is because we hold on to old, painful memories. When we suppress we hold on, so any pain which we suppress, we sustain in our unconscious minds and in the cellular memory of our body. So in many ways, every illness is an opportunity for transformation.

I encourage my clients to forgive their enemies or people who are putting them down, as forgiveness releases the divine energy held in our cells and frees us to be whole and healed. So remember: it is time now to forgive. It is time now for transformation.

4
PHYSICAL HEALTH

ARTHRITIS

Q: *Could you tell me a bit more about arthritis? I have pains in my hands and hips, and the pain seems to be worse after certain foods or when I am stressed at work. Is there a connection?*

A: Yes there is a connection! But first let me begin by defining the different types of arthritis, and some of the possible causes. The word "arthritis" means inflammation of the joint. In osteoarthritis, degeneration begins with the joint itself and is usually caused by a calcium deficiency within the bones, or by a previous injury. Rheumatoid arthritis is not a disease of the skeletal structure like arthritis. Rather it is a disease of the immune system, known as an auto-immune disease, where the white blood cells attack their own host body cells, ie the joint in the case of rheumatoid arthritis. Osteoporosis (porous bones) is more common in women over 50, and can lead to easy fractures. In many cases, the problems stem from calcium not being absorbed adequately. This mal-absorption may result from a number of contributory factors, including:

- **Excess alcohol (red wine), tea, coffee and cocoa (these are all acidic to the body and inhibit the adequate absorption of calcium)**
- **Lack of hydrochloric acid in the diet (practice the Hay Diet to prevent this)**
- **Intake of too many acid-forming foods (especially too much meat) which inhibit calcium absorption**
- **Hormone imbalance**
- **Insufficient exercise (by simply walking more frequently, you could raise calcium levels in the body by 2% or more)**
- **Over-use of sugar in the diet**
- **Too much stress in your life, increasing the need for calcium**
- **Over-consumption of dairy products (dairy products provide calcium but not the magnesium which the body requires to absorb the calcium).**

So your diet may indeed be exacerbating your problem. Here is a list of which foods to avoid and which to eat:

• **Foods to Avoid**	• **Foods to Eat**
X Wheat (if allergic) & excess dairy products	✓ Wheat-free grains like brown rice, millet & spelt
X Sugar & foods which contain sugar	✓ Raw and cooked dark green vegetables
X Non-organic salt	✓ Sea salt
X Excess tea	✓ Herbal teas, especially green tea which is a great detoxant to the body
X Alcohol, soft drinks, coffee & tap water	✓ White meat, fish & eggs
X Citrus fruits	✓ Fresh, raw fruits, especially bananas & pineapple (but not citrus)
X Artificial additives & preservatives	✓ Spring water, fruit juice (not citrus), vegetable juice
X The "Nightshade" family: potatoes (except juice), tomatoes, peppers & aubergines	✓ Raw potato juice *
	✓ Nuts & seeds

* wash a medium organic potato, cut into thin slices, and place in a large jar filled with spring water. Let stand overnight, remove slices, and drink first thing in the morning.

You should exercise regularly and practice yoga to help reduce stress levels in the body: too much stress can also make your arthritis worse. In her book "You Can Heal Your Life", Louise Hay states that arthritis comes from a constant pattern of criticism – criticism of the self and also of other people.

Such people can also be perfectionists. If this sounds like you, try these daily affirmations:

"I am love. I now choose to love and approve of myself. I see others with love."

Because there are so many factors at play with arthritis – diet, lifestyle, genetics, allergies and so on – I cannot really recommend any specific homeopathic remedies: you should consult with a practitioner for an individual consultation which is tailored to your specific circumstances. You might also consider adding essential fatty acids to your diet (available from any good health store), and digestive enzymes if the Hay Diet is not practical for you.

ASTHMA

Asthma can be inherited, and may be caused by an unknown allergy. It can be aggravated by infections such as colds, and by anxiety. During an asthma attack, the lung airways (or bronchi) contract, and a build up of mucus occurs in the tubes. The patient experiences tightness in the chest, accompanied by breathlessness and wheezing. In acute phases it can be frightening, and in the case of a severe serious attack, medical help should be sought immediately.

Asthma is more common in boys, typically starting from 3 years as opposed to 8 years with girls. If allergies such as hay fever run in your family, then your child is more at risk. Babies who have recurrent colds, catarrh or eczema are more likely to develop asthma as they grow older. There are several homeopathic remedies that can help with asthma, including Aconite, Arsenicum, Chamomilla, Ipecac, Nat Sulph and Pulsatilla. For a complete cure, however, a constitutional treatment by a qualified homeopath is essential - although this can take time.

Asthma attacks can be triggered by straightforward allergies – for example to cat hair – but they can also be caused by emotional upsets and stressful situations. The asthmatic child can be highly-strung, nervous and sensitive. Coughing and wheezing can also be caused by viral infections such as colds and bronchitis, and by genetic lung diseases such as cystic fibrosis.

Common triggers for asthma are listed below, and should be avoided if possible.

- **Cigarette smoke**
- **Air pollution (eg dust mites, house dust, molds, car exhaust fumes, feather pillows etc)**
- **Grass, flower and tree pollen**
- **Strenuous exercise, especially in cold, dry air**
- **Food additives, especially yellow dyes, sodium benzoate and sulphites**
- **Colds and cold viruses**
- **Emotional stress**
- **Aspirin (this most common medication can cause asthmatic flare-ups)**
- **Perfumes**

- **Aerosol products such as hairspray, furniture polish etc.**

Practical tips for minimising asthma attacks are as follows:

- **Keep the child's bedroom as clean as possible: regularly dust with a damp cloth.**
- **Drink plenty of pure, filtered water. Water helps to keep mucus secretions thin and loose, preventing them from becoming dry, sticky and difficult to clear from the lungs.**
- **A diet low in magnesium is associated with wheezing, so eat good sources of magnesium such as wholegrains, soya beans, shrimp and green, leafy vegetables.**
- **Fish oils from fatty fish such as mackerel, salmon, sardines and tuna are good for combating asthma: you can also take fish oil supplements.**
- **Onions, asparagus, turnips, cabbage and brussel sprouts appear to be beneficial for all kinds of respiratory disorders, including asthma.**
- **Try the following fresh juice blend: 4 oz/120g of raspberries, 4 oz/120g of strawberries and 1 orange. Take 120ml / day.**
- **Sunflower seeds are beneficial for asthmatics. Sprinkle ground-up seeds over natural yoghurt and honey, and into breakfast cereal.**
- **Emotional stress releasing massage once a week using 10 drops of lavender and roman chamomile essential oils in 10mls carrier oil.**
- **Yoga breathing methods strengthen the lungs and diaphragm. Get your child to place his hands on his abdomen and breathe in slowly, feeling his stomach pushing out. Ask the child to hold this for a moment, then breathe out slowly.**
- **Plunging the feet into a hot footbath can help to ease an attack.**
- **Reflexology point: try massaging the reflex area between the big toe and second toe on both feet.**

BROKEN LEG

Q: *My 72 year old mother slipped in the bathroom last week and broke her leg in several places. Can you suggest any homeopathic remedies that could help in her healing process? She has just been discharged from hospital with a plaster of Paris, and is very impatient at the moment.*

A: I do sympathise - it's difficult when you see a loved one immobilized by something like a broken leg. But your Mum needs to be patient with herself whilst her body heals: rest has a vital role to play in helping the body to recover. In response to your question, yes, homeopathic remedies can be of assistance in accelerating the healing process of her fracture, and they can also help to prevent deep vein thrombosis. Below is a list of recommended remedies: you should be able to buy a 30 potency in local health shops, pharmacies or dedicated homeopathic pharmacies. The remedies described are also useful for other broken bones, not just leg fractures. Remember, if you are in any doubt about whether a bone is broken, you should always seek medical advice – an X-ray will confirm the situation.

ARNICA has a profound effect on circulation, and helps to stop bleeding. It aids healing, reduces swelling at the injured site, and is also useful for pain relief. Arnica is a major remedy in helping to prevent deep vein thrombosis, where its action is to dissolve the blood clot, especially if the patient is bedridden. It is also useful to use after a stroke. Always assess any injury before using Arnica, as it may mask a fracture by reducing the pain and swelling.

ACONITE is a good remedy to use for fright, fear or shock after an injury, when the vital force of the person has been disturbed. Symptoms may include pale skin, breaking into cold sweats, and the desire to urinate more frequently than usual. The patient may also be very restless in sleep or even be prone to nightmares.

SYMPHYTUM is also known as "knitbone", and does exactly what it says on the tin: it helps the bone to knit together! You should not use this remedy until the broken bone is set in the right place.

CAL PHOS should be used as a tissue salt in a 6x potency. Calcium and phosphorous are the two main minerals needed for building up healthy bones.

Use this remedy after the broken bone has properly knitted together, and give daily until fully healed. Cal Phos is a good remedy for people with weak or brittle bones that are prone to factures.

Take one of the above remedies twice daily for two weeks. Remedies can be taken together if required. Finally, a reminder that it is perfectly safe to take homeopathic remedies alongside orthodox medicines.

CANCER

Q: *Can you explain why it is that some people get cancer and others not? Does it mean also that because my mother (still living) had breast cancer that I have a higher risk of getting it?*

A: Whether we like it or not, we all have the potential to develop cancer! TB was one of the main illnesses of the 19th century, and cancer is one of the main ones of this century. In her book "The Bodymind Workbook", Debbie Shapiro explores how the mind and body work together. According to her, cancer can develop when the immune system becomes suppressed. It appears that cancer cells are developing in our body all the time, but that they are normally destroyed by our immune system.

So what is it that causes the changes in the cells to make them become malignant? Could it be that because the body has grown so used to the abnormality in terms of thought patterns and attitudes, it does not recognise the difference when those thought patterns become malignant? Many argue that cancer can be the result of years of inner conflict, guilt, hurt, grief, resentment, confusion or tension surrounding personal issues. They say that it can also be connected to feelings of hopelessness, inadequacy and self-rejection. Cancer has even been called "acceptable suicide". It is as if the deeply embedded resentments or conflicts eventually eat away at the body itself.

The "cancer" personality that has emerged after years of research is one that is very loving, supportive and kind, but which simultaneously represses personal feelings, is long-suffering and has a low sense of self-esteem. When we give so much to others, we are often putting their needs ahead of our own and are not giving to ourselves – not really loving or honouring ourselves. The cancer-prone personality is often the "rock" of the family, the one who carries all the problems but never complains.

So to come back to your question, in my family there is a history of heart disease, and several relatives died from it in their early 40's. But I don't dwell on the fear of a heart attack or even death as I approach my mid 40's. My approach is to empower myself and to live life to its fullest, and this is what you should do too. Let your good intentions create positive experiences for you. Learn to give and receive love easily. Express your feelings and don't bottle them up. Boost your immune system with natural medicine, eat a healthy diet and exercise often. Most importantly, learn to have fun and enjoy life. Have a regular mammogram, and believe you are healthy before you get your results!

CANDIDA

Q: *I keep suffering from feelings of bloatedness and tiredness. I also have small white spots in my mouth. A friend reckons I may have candida. Can you tell me more about candida and how to treat it?*

A: From the description of your symptoms, it does sound like you have candida. You are not alone: it is an all too common condition, and I see a very high percentage of clients who suffer from it.

Candida (also called thrush) is a yeast-like organism that can thrive in the gastro-intestinal tract when the levels of beneficial bacteria are low. It may cause tiny white spots in the mouth, anal itching, feelings of bloatedness and tiredness after eating, indigestion, and a craving for sugar. Potential causes include:

- **Over-consumption of sugar or yeast products**
- **Repeated courses of antibiotics**
- **Steroids**
- **Birth control pills**
- **Stress.**

If the immune system is too weak to overcome it, candida can spread throughout the body. In extreme cases it can cause damage to the gut wall, ie "leaky gut", which can eventually weaken the immune system still more, giving rise to fatigue, depression, headaches, impaired memory, digestive problems, recurrent vaginitis and cystitis, PMT, irritability, hypothyroidism (underactive thyroid) and hypoglycaemia (low blood sugar). It also commonly causes food, drug and chemical sensitivities.

Your diet plays a critical role in helping to treat candida. Here's a list of foods to avoid and foods to eat:

• **Foods to Avoid**	• **Foods to Eat**
X Cheeses, including cottage & cream cheese	✓ Meat, fish, fowl & shellfish
X Bread made with yeast	✓ Eggs & butter
X Cakes	✓ Brown rice, oats & millet
X Pitta breads & buns	✓ Fresh vegetables
X Marmite & Bovril	✓ Spelt bread, rye crispbreads, chapattis
X Sugar & foods which contain sugar	✓ Fresh nuts (not peanuts) & seeds
X Pickled & smoked meat & fish	✓ Cold pressed vegetable oils
X Fruit (first 3 to 4 weeks only)	✓ Fresh herbs & spices, especially garlic
X Mushrooms	✓ Snacks: rice cakes & oat cakes
X Soy sauce & stock cubes	✓ Soya / Rice / Goat's milk
X Vinegar, pickles & ketchup	✓ Herb teas
X Beer, wine, cider & spirits	

In my experience, I have found that the homeopathic medicines Lycopodium and Thuja taken together really help in the treatment of candida. Lycopodium reduces the craving for the sweet things that feed the yeast, and helps to detox the liver. It is important to cut sugar out of the diet, as it feeds the yeast. Thuja acts as a blood cleanser and helps to support the correct bacterial flora that aid digestion in the gut. Successful treatment of candida can take as long as three months, so you need to be patient: take the remedies for two weeks, and then leave a gap of two weeks, before you start taking them again.

If you would like to know more, then I would recommend you read the book "Candida Albicans" by Leon Chaitlow.

CHILDHOOD FEVERS

Q: *My two year old daughter gets repeated fevers. Is there any homeopathic remedy that could help to bring down her temperature?*

A:Yes, there are indeed a number of homeopathic remedies that can help your daughter. But before going any further, some general advice about fevers: if you are in any doubt as to the seriousness of the fever, you should consult a registered health professional! Take especial caution if the temperature remains above 40°C for more than 24 hours, particularly if there is a history of convulsions, or if the child is under six months old.

Normal body temperatures are as follows: oral 37°C (98.6°F), rectal 37.5°C (99.6°F) and from the armpit 36.5°C (97.6°F). Infants may have a slightly raised temperature in the evening. This is normal and is not necessarily a cause for alarm. Fever is one of nature's ways of helping our bodies to fight off disease (unless the fever is extremely high or complicated by other factors), so, in at least some respects, it is beneficial and should not necessarily be a cause for worry.

Fevers in childhood often precede – and / or accompany – conditions like earache, respiratory problems, contagious diseases (eg mumps, chicken pox etc), teething or flu. So when you are looking for the correct homeopathic remedy, it is not only the fever that needs to be observed. Two factors are key: first, what kind of fever, and secondly how your child behaves when ill. Also, the aim is to cure the child, not just to reduce the fever. A positive change after a remedy may not always take the form of bringing the fever down straightaway – the child may feel better in him/herself, or their appetite may return, for example, with the fever gradually coming down. If your child falls asleep shortly after taking a remedy, this may be a good sign and often means the fever should then improve. So here are the three most useful homeopathic remedies for childhood fevers:

ACONITE: Sudden, rapid onset of symptoms, accompanied by high fever. Worse for exposure to cold, dry weather. Child is very restless, anxious and fearful. Child is dry, hot and thirsty. Rapid pulse. Fear often accompanies an Aconite fever, or the fever may start after fear or a shock or fright to the system.

BELLADONNA: Sudden, rapid onset of symptoms, accompanied by high fever. Bright red, flushed face. Dilated, shiny pupils, eyes red. Skin burning hot, can feel steamy. Hot head but cold feet. Irritable. Throbbing headache. May have no sense of thirst.

FERR PHOS: Fever with pink cheeks and a pale face. Useful at the beginning of the fever. Onset of fever is not as rapid or extreme as Aconite or Belladonna.

Choose the remedy which most closely matches your child's symptoms, and give a 30 potency every 30 to 60 minutes. If after 3 doses the fever has improved but tends to keep coming back quickly, repeat as needed for a few more doses. As the child improves, increase the length of time between doses to two hourly, four hourly and then am / pm. But to reiterate, if you are in any doubt, you should consult a registered health professional.

CHILDHOOD SLEEPING PROBLEMS

Q: *My 8 year old daughter is not sleeping very well at present. She wakes up several times a night worrying that a robber is going to break in. In order to get some sleep, I am allowing her to sleep with me and my husband in our bed, but now it's me who can't sleep! So can you make any suggestions on getting her to sleep the night through again?*

A: Your daughter appears to be a very sensitive child. I have come across many similar children in my clinics with similar symptoms to your daughter. I wonder if she has seen or read anything that has upset her? There has been an awful lot of focus on negativity in the media with the Madeleine McCann case recently, and I wonder if this is what has affected her. Unfortunately, focussing on negativity only causes more negativity – that is one of the reasons why there is so much negativity in our world these days. The media – television, radio, newspapers, movies, magazines and books – all contribute to this focus, especially when they portray bad news – sadly, bad news sells!

So what can you do to help your daughter? Firstly, reassure her at all times that she is safe, and talk about the extreme abduction of Madeline (especially if you think this might be the root of the problem). Aconite is the first homeopathic remedy you should consider giving her. This remedy is wonderfully effective for ailments arising from shock or bad news. Shock can be stored in the body's cellular memory, and can result in the following symptoms:

- **Beating heart and palpitations**
- **Person is very nervous, jumpy and startled easily**
- **Goes to the toilet frequently.**

If Aconite does not shift your daughter's symptoms, you could try giving her the homeopathic remedies Lycopodium and Nat Mur. In all cases, use a 30 potency, and give her the remedies morning and evening for two weeks only, and then take a break for two weeks to allow her body to do its own healing. These remedies will help with your daughter's subconscious and conscious fears about robbers and her worry that something bad might happen. They will also help her to be more confident in herself and to trust more.

It might be a good idea for you to observe her TV viewing, as sometimes a child's imagination is so vivid it can be detrimental to their well-being. The behaviour of some children often mirrors the emotions and feelings of the adults around them – so be aware of your own emotions! Try and focus on positive things. Remember, if you only focus on positive things, in time our

world becomes more positive. Good luck and sweet dreams!

"Always listen to children."

CONSTIPATION

Q: *I suffer from constipation. I am in my fifties and eat a fairly high fibre diet, yet I can get no relief. I would be grateful for any advice.*

A: The bowel is made up of the large intestine, which is five feet long, and the small intestine which is 20 feet long – so isn't it amazing that anything finds its way out of the body at all?! Although constipation is not an illness in itself, it can be a symptom that something is wrong. There are many potential causes:

- **Poor constitution (I can usually see this in the eyes by using iridology)**
- **Inadequate or unsuitable diet – this includes intolerance to certain food groups, the most common being dairy and wheat products**
- **Stress in one's life**
- **Side effects from medication.**

Constipation can lead to a general state of lowered health, for sluggish stools can lead to people who are sluggish both physically and mentally. Indeed, I often think of the bowel as our second brain. If you have a clean bowel, then you have a clearer head. Constipation can lead to bad breath, body odour and haemorrhoids. In more chronic cases, it can result in varicose veins, headaches, insomnia, diverticulitis (inflammation of the pouches of the colon) and even bowel cancer.

From an emotional perspective, constipation is a holding on, a tightening of the muscles such that elimination cannot take place. This may be due to a fear or a worry that something bad may happen. In my experience, people are much more likely to suffer from constipation when they are facing financial problems, relationship conflicts or travelling abroad. These are all times when we may feel insecure and ungrounded, leading to a desire to hold on to everything as it is, and not let uncertain change come upon us. I wonder if any of this rings a bell with you?

To help combat constipation, try the following steps:

- **Drink eight to ten glasses of filtered water a day**

- **Cut back on the tea and coffee (a maximum of two cups a day) – drink herbal teas instead**
- **Try "Lepicol" psyllium husks each morning: it's a natural plant fibre with acidophyllodus which aids elimination**
- **Cut out white bread, milk and cheese, and change to breads made from high fibre grains (rotate different grains in your diet). Milk, chocolate and cheese can block the bowel in some people, as the colon finds them indigestible. Switch to nut milks, oat milk or soya milks, and again, rotate.**
- **Eat six vegetable and two fruit portions a day, preferably some raw to add more bulk and fibre.**

Finally, trust more in the flow of life. When you trust, you go with the synchronicity of life rather than being too controlling. Let go of your fears and trust that everything will be OK. This also means learning to play more and have fun, expressing yourself more freely, and accepting and being at peace with whatever life throws at you. Next time you find yourself worrying about something, or trying to be too controlling, say to yourself "I trust", and watch the changes happen.

CYSTITIS

Q: *Can you suggest a homeopathic remedy for cystitis? I broke up with my long-term boyfriend a few months ago, and since then I keep getting recurrent infections.*

A: Cystitis is an acute bladder infection, most often caused by a bacterial infection. The bladder is the collecting chamber in the body which stores waste fluid until it is released as urine. The bladder also helps in the cleansing and releasing of negative emotions. Signs and symptoms of cystitis include:

- **Burning pains during urination**
- **Strong desire to pass urine but with little success.**

Research has shown that cases of cystitis are more common during and after the break up of a relationship. During this potentially traumatic time, if negative emotions are not being expressed – in the form of things like hurt pride, anger, fear of being alone, feelings of loss and rejection and so on – then these repressed emotions may begin to accumulate and cause intense irritation and frustration. So the upset caused by the break up with your boyfriend may be the maintaining cause of your imbalance, contributing to the recurrent cystitis. The remedies described below should help: and talking your feelings through with friends and family will also be of assistance.

CANTHARIS: Urine is scalding. Desperate urge to go but with very little urine passed. Urine cloudy in colour.

CAUSTICUM: Burning sensation passing urine. Involuntary passing of urine on coughing. Retention of urine.

SARSAPARILLA: Pain is worst at the close of urination. Scalding urine.

Practical advice for cystitis is as follows:

- **Don't hold on when you need to spend a penny.**
- **Avoid using scented bubble baths, soaps and wipes as the chemicals they contain can be irritating.**

- **Drink 8 to 10 glasses of filtered water daily.**
- **Cranberry juice (sugar free) helps produce hippuric acid in the urine which acidifies the urinary tract and inhibits the growth of bacteria.**
- **Raspberries and avocados are helpful foods as they reduce the proliferation of unfriendly bacteria in the bladder.**
- **Celery and parsley are natural diuretics. Garlic and onions are also antibiotic in action.**
- **Drink the following fresh juice blend: 1 apple, 1 pear, 3 fl oz / 90 ml of water. Take 5 fl oz / 150 ml daily.**
- **During an attack of cystitis, eliminate sugar, refined carbohydrates, dried fruits and foods which contain yeast (eg bread, croissants, Marmite, vinegar and pickles) from your diet. Sugar feeds the yeast, which can contribute to cystitis.**
- **If you are given antibiotics for the infection, be sure to take B Complex vitamin, and the homeopathic remedy Thuja 30 potency, which you should take am and pm for two weeks, to help cleanse the blood and prevent candida.**
- **Add 10 drops of sandalwood essential oil to your bath.**

EAR INFECTIONS

Q: *My four year old son keeps on getting repeated ear infections. He has now had his sixth antibiotic and still the infection keeps recurring. I'm at my wits end! Can you help? Are there any homeopathic remedies that might help?*

A:Yes, homeopathic remedies could help, not alone to build up your son's immune system, but also to treat the symptoms and the cause of the infection. But you should also consider your son's diet, and look seriously at the treatment he has had so far – if he's on his sixth course of antibiotics, the current approach is clearly not working! If the infection is viral, then antibiotics will not be effective – in fact they can be more suppressive in nature. Also, try keeping your son off dairy products (ie milk, cheese, chocolate etc), and switch to goat's, soya or rice milk. Milk can produce too much mucus, and this may be what is clogging up your son's lymphatic system. His ears may then try to discharge the disharmony within the body and so become infected.

Try the following homeopathic remedies, remembering to choose the one which most closely matches his symptoms. Take a 30 potency morning and evening for 2 weeks, then break for 2 weeks to give his body the chance to heal. If this is unsuccessful, then I would recommend you consult with your local homeopath to get him assessed in greater detail.

PULSATILLA: Ear ache may come and go with no pattern. Child is weepy and irritable, but better for affection and sympathy. Child feels more comfortable if the room is cool or when outdoors. Itching deep in ears. Thick, bland, offensive discharge. Cracking sensation in ears.

MERCURY: Pain from the ears may extend to the throat and mouth. Discharge is yellow and occasionally blood streaked. Glands in the face and neck may be swollen and hard. Child is likely to be thirsty and sweaty, and have lots of saliva that smells bad.

HEPAR SULPH: Pus has begun to build up in the ears. Sore throat may also be present, with a yellow-green discharge. Pain is sharp, and the child feels cross and needs lots of warmth.

BELLADONNA: Symptoms of ear ache come on very quickly. Ear ache is intensely painful, the ear throbs and looks red. Temperature may be high.

ECZEMA

Q: *My 2 year old daughter has terrible eczema, oozing and so, so itchy. Could homeopathy help her? The steroid cream the doctor gave her seems only to help temporarily, and she has had repeated chest infections. She has been given numerous antibiotics too, but they don't seem to help. Please help!*

A: It is difficult as a Mum to stand by and watch your child suffer in such discomfort from eczema. First, let me explain what eczema is:

Eczema is a skin condition in which the skin is irritated or inflamed. You can't catch eczema, and the exact cause is not fully understood, although it can be genetic. In passing, I should also mention that I have seen kids who had no eczema prior to vaccinations and who developed it after the jabs – but I will leave this conjecture open, until further research becomes more widely available. The symptoms of eczema are red, dry and itchy skin, small white blisters, particularly on the hands and feet, and scaly areas in places that are scratched frequently.

From long experience of treating eczema in my clinics, I have found that the following can help to aid the child's recovery:

- **Cut out cow's milk and switch to goat's or soya milk. Many children find cow's milk indigestible and can build up an intolerance to it. Remember too that breast is best, and next comes goat's milk.**
- **Change your washing powder to an eco-friendly, non bio brand.**
- **Colloidal silver solution massaged into the skin can help to ease the itch and prevent infection, and is available at your local health shop.**
- **Remember that the skin is a channel of elimination. If it is not supported in its excretory functions, then suppression – through the usage of such treatments as steroid creams – may push the disorder further into the body, and result in problems arising elsewhere in the body, for example in the form of asthma.**
- **Consult with a professional homeopath. In my experience, no two cases are alike, meaning each patient requires a different, individually tailored prescription to help boost their immune system and fight the eczema.**

Depending on the maintaining cause – be it genetic, allergies, low immune system or whatever – I believe that each child can override their eczema. But it can take months (the skin regenerates every 3 months) – so patience is required, and often things will get worse before they get better.

HEAD LICE

Q: *My kids keep getting head lice. I don't like chemicals but may have to resort to them if this continues! Have you any advice on natural treatments that work?*

A: As the mother of 4 children, I know all about your dilemma! I have written about this problem in the past, and having tried numerous natural approaches, I have recently discovered something quick and easy compared to other natural treatments, and which really works.

Head lice are small six legged insects that live on the human scalp and in the hair. They cannot fly, jump or swim, but can be spread through close head contact or via brushes, combs etc. They only infest humans, so you cannot catch them from animals. Head lice feed by sucking blood through the scalp. The female produces eggs which are very firmly glued on to hair shafts close to the scalp, and the nits hatch out every 7 to 10 days. Some children seem to be more susceptible to the problem, but the reasons for this are not fully understood.

So what is the name of the product I've recently discovered? Well, it's a product called "Nitty Gritty" – it's an aromatherapy oil made by Mums, and I have found it to be most effective with my own kids. I dislike most conventional treatments, as they typically contain insecticides which are inherently toxic. It is interesting to note that in the USA, insecticides are not allowed to be labelled as safe, because of their toxicity. There is particular concern over organophosphates and organochlorines, some of which have been found to be carcinogenic.

Several health authorities in the UK advise against the use of insecticide-based lotions except as a last resort, as the lice can become immune to them, and the lotions can poison not just the child's body but also the environment.

Nitty Gritty natural aromatherapy oil is to be left in the hair for 20 minutes, then combed with a fine-tooth nit comb. This needs to be done weekly to prevent re-infestation. It is available from local health shops and pharmacies. Some final words of advice: remember to keep the child's brush / comb separate, do not share it with other people, and wash it regularly to prevent cross infection. Nitty Gritty really worked for my kids, so good luck! You can find out more at www.nittygritty.co.uk.

HIGH BLOOD PRESSURE

Q: *I suffer from high blood pressure, and would be grateful for any advice you could give me on treating it naturally. I would love to come off my medication and have my blood pressure stable.*

A: Blood pressure is controlled by the brain, the kidneys and the adrenal glands, plus the autonomic nervous system. Our blood pressure can alter during the day by as much as 30 points, and will always rise when we are pressured, nervous, anxious or rushing for an appointment. Never accept a single reading as being an accurate reflection of your average blood pressure; you should have at least three readings.

Most people I treat for hypertension (ie high blood pressure) would typically suffer from excessive emotional tension. The causes may include a deep-seated fear or a lack of trust – a feeling that we are in constant danger and need to be on our guard at all times. This may be due to a traumatic experience in the past. Remember, a long-standing emotional problem can be hidden in your body's cells. Our bodies have a cellular memory, and sometimes that memory needs to be released. The following advice may be useful in helping to lower your blood pressure:

- **Follow a mostly vegetarian diet (avoid red meat, and if possible eat fish only).**
- **Juice fasting: one day a week just drink vegetable juice instead of eating food. One cup of freshly-made vegetable juice contains 2g of potassium and helps to reduce blood pressure.**
- **Eat garlic: 15g per day (one to four cloves) is said to help prevent heart disease and strokes.**
- **Eat a high-fibre diet: whole grains, pulses, raw nuts and seeds including sunflower and flax seeds. Millet, oats, spelt and oat-bran make an ideal breakfast. Buckwheat lowers blood pressure thanks to its beneficial effects on blood vessel walls.**
- **Oily fish lowers blood pressure.**
- **Avoid sugar and refined carbohydrates (ie white flour, white bread, white rice, cornstarch and everything made from them).**

- **Avoid all processed foods.**
- **Avoid caffeine, alcohol and cigarettes.**
- **Say the following affirmation daily to help release any emotional issues: "I joyously release the past. I am at peace."**

Often, hypertension can be the result of repressed anger: people are sweet and wholesome on the outside but seething with anger on the inside. I use a 30 potency of the homeopathic remedy Lachesis, one twice daily for two weeks, to treat this, and have had a lot of success with this remedy.

Keep monitoring your blood pressure on a regular basis. Send love to your enemy, as this changes cells to become more love-based, helping to release anger and hence lower your blood pressure. Go on – try it, it works!

HIGH CHOLESTEROL

Q: *I've had tests which reveal my blood cholesterol levels are up. I've been on a low fat diet for a year. The next step is medication to lower the levels, but I don't really want to go down this route. I feel a bit pressurised to do something, as there is a history of heart disease in my family. Any advice would be gratefully received.*

A: This high cholesterol problem is becoming all too common. I see several clients a week asking me the same question. It can be very disillusioning after being on a healthy diet for a year to still have high cholesterol.

We know that fatty foods - ie animal fats (sausages, pork, bacon, ham etc), ice cream, cheese, fried foods etc - encourage fatty plaques to form in the blood that can block arteries. But did you also know that from an emotional perspective, the heart in our body represents love, whilst our blood represents joy? Our hearts lovingly pump joy throughout our bodies. When we deny ourselves love and joy, the heart shrivels and becomes cold. As a result, the blood gets sluggish and we may find ourselves with high cholesterol, high blood pressure, anaemia, angina and heart attacks. But the heart does not "attack" us. We get so caught up in the soap operas and dramas that we create in our lives, that we forget to notice the small joys that surround us. We spend years squeezing all the joy out of our blood and heart, and this literally has its consequences in our bodies.

So my advice to you is to take a long, reflective look at your life. Take time out, starting today, and try to appreciate all the small joys in your life. Do the things that give you more joy and happiness, like gardening, painting, dancing and so on. Create inner sanctuary time for yourself, and maybe join a yoga, tai chi or Pilates class. Be kind to yourself: treat yourself to a facial, massage, pedicure or manicure. Change your diet further if you need to (you may need to consult with a nutritionist). Above all, have a sense of humour and laugh as much as possible. Go and see comedy shows and lighten up your life, and don't forget to enjoy the journey.

The following affirmation, repeated twice daily, can also help to bring more joy to the blood and hence reduce the cholesterol.

"I tune into the love, joy, peace, happiness and laughter within me. I am at peace with myself. I accept myself."

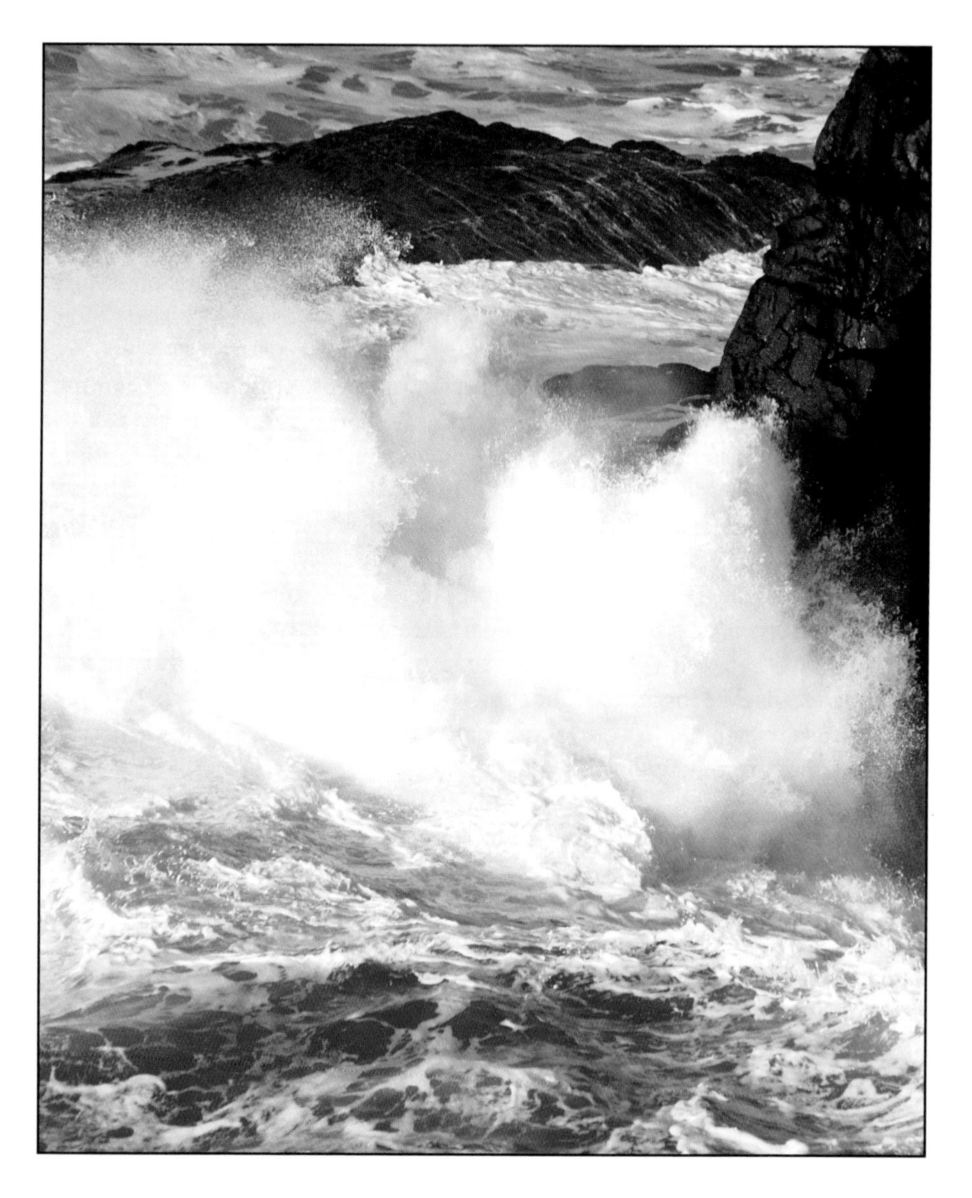

"It takes as much energy to create sickness as to create health." ~ *Shaun de Warren*

INDIGESTION & HEARTBURN

Q: *I frequently suffer from indigestion and heartburn. It's worse after I eat food, and I was wondering if you could suggest anything to help cure it.*

A: Indigestion is a very broad term that refers to virtually any problem relating to digesting food. Most commonly, it refers to heartburn, gas or distension of the stomach. When heartburn occurs, the oesophagus (wind pipe) or stomach is irritated by too much acid, either from the foods eaten or from the digestive acids that are secreted to digest them. Problems can also be caused by underproduction of hydrochloric acid, which leads to an inability to break down food and hence to indigestion. The body may slightly regurgitate the food and acids, thereby creating a burning sensation in the middle of the chest. Heartburn is an uncomfortable condition, but symptoms like it are there to let you know that something is out of balance.

It is sadly the case that, for many reasons, we do not digest all the food we eat. Indeed, you might say that "you are what you assimilate" rather than "you are what you eat"! But even this "truism" is not the full story, as it focuses too narrowly on food alone. If you are what your body takes in, then what about what you inhale? (not just fresh air, but also cigarette smoke and car fumes). Or what your skin absorbs? Or what your mind thinks? If we take on all this and more, it is certainly understandable why so many people suffer from indigestion! The point here is that the cause of your problems may well be from factors other than digestion! Perhaps you are over sensitive. Or you cannot "stomach" all that is going on around you.

As we get older (from our late 30's), our bodies can get burdened by the process of digestion. What we could eat in our 20's suddenly becomes indigestible. This often happens because our bodies do not produce enough digestive enzymes. So try following the advice below and watch the healing take place:

- **Eat your food slowly, with approximately 40 chews per portion of food. Also eat small meals, four hourly if necessary, to help the body to break down the food more efficiently.**
- **Don't drink water, milk or alcohol with your food. Wait 20 minutes before and after. Liquids can dilute the acid in our stomachs which is there to help break down our food.**

- **Don't eat late at night. Food eaten late at night takes longer to digest. The liver and digestive organs like a rest too, so let them have one!**
- **Practice the Hay Diet: separate your proteins (eg meat, fish, eggs, cheese etc) from your starches (eg potatoes, bread, rice, pasta etc). Neutrals like salads and vegetables can be eaten with either the starches or proteins. Hydrochloric acid breaks down proteins, whilst digestive enzymes break down starches: the two combined together can make it more difficult to break down these foods, and hence lead to indigestion. Birds in nature actually follow the Hay Diet, and separate their proteins from their starches!**
- **If you eat too many acid-type foods, ie white bread, meat, cheese, coffee, tea, alcohol etc, then you should try eating more alkaline foods like raw vegetables and salads, and just under-ripe fruit (over-ripe fruits are acidic). 40% of your diet should be raw-based to help secrete digestive enzymes to aid digestion (salads, juices, raw vegetables etc). Fresh papaya and pineapple eaten 15 minutes before a meal can also enhance the production of the enzymes that aid the digestive process.**
- **Raw, unpeeled almonds are the only nuts that are alkaline: they help to neutralise an overacidic stomach and are excellent for getting rid of heartburn.**
- **Avoid heartburn hotel: as you are most likely aware, certain foods can irritate the lining of the stomach and oesophagus, and should be avoided: these include coffee and acidic fruits like tomatoes.**
- **Cut out white bread, as it is a low energy food and you may find it harder to tolerate as you get older.**

You could also try the homeopathic remedy Nat Mur 30 potency, one twice daily for 2 weeks. This can alleviate heartburn and help with the assimilation and absorption of nutrients into the body. There are several other remedies that are excellent for treating heartburn and indigestion, so I would recommend you consult with your local homeopath for a solution that is tailored to your individual circumstances.

INSOMNIA

Time is not the only great healer: sleep is too! Sleep helps our body cells to rejuvenate and heal, but a lack of sleep can leave us feeling tired, depressed and low.

I treat many patients with insomnia, and it is a surprisingly common complaint: as many as 15 – 25% of adults regularly suffer from it. Whilst some insomniacs have difficulty falling asleep, others wake up frequently and have problems getting back to sleep or staying asleep.

Insomnia may suggest a deep fear of letting go and surrendering. When we sleep, we are in a vulnerable and surrendered state, and the inability to sleep may indicate chronic tension, fear and anxiety. Ongoing insomnia can also indicate a severe lack of trust. The thymus gland is closely connected to sleep, and in turn the thymus is connected to the energy of the heart. Thus insomnia is often related to our ability to love ourselves, to trust love and therefore to trust life.

Perhaps the best way to determine whether you are getting enough sleep each night is to see how you feel upon waking. You should be rested and refreshed. If you are not, then the following remedies can help (remember to choose the symptoms that most closely relate to your body). Use a 30 potency half an hour before bedtime and then again at bedtime. Repeat hourly if necessary.

ARSENICUM: Sleeplessness due to anxiety. Great restlessness, constant tossing and turning. Cannot drop off, could be awake to 2 – 3 am. Likes to have head raised on pillows. Dreams are full of death, sorrow and fire. Can be oversensitive and fastidious, wanting everything in its own place. Constant worrying like a hamster on a wheel, and cannot make it stop.

COFFEA: Sleeps until 3 am, thereafter only dozing. Sleeplessness due to over-activity of the brain, lots of ideas churning around in the head. Memory overactive before midnight, also leading to sleeplessness.

NUX VOMICA: Falls asleep long before bedtime then wakes up at 2 am and cannot sleep. Sleepless from rush of ideas to the head. Falls asleep at daybreak and then feels weak and tired upon rising. Can suffer from anger and impatience. Can be headstrong and stubborn, with anxiety on waking in the morning.

AURUM: Awake all night, or falls asleep and wakes up between 4 – 5 am. May moan and cry out in sleep. May suffer from depression with feelings of worthlessness and guilt. Takes life too seriously with forsaken feelings. Oversensitive to being contradicted. Can be a workaholic with feelings of too much responsibility. Wants to be the best. Aurum is made from gold, and silver and bronze are never good enough in this person's eyes: they are always going for gold, and this puts a lot of pressure on them.

Here are some useful tips to help with insomnia:

- **Before bedtime, take a warm bath with a few drops of relaxing aromatherapy oils such as clary sage or roman chamomile.**
- **Avoid caffeinated products such as coffee, black tea, colas etc. Nicotine in cigarettes is also a stimulant that can keep you awake at night.**
- **Despite folklore that has long suggested that warm milk helps people sleep, research has shown that it is rarely helpful. In fact, non-fat and low-fat milk can actually stimulate activity in the brain!**
- **Bedrooms should be used for sleeping and not for stressful activities like paying bills or doing work.**
- **Finally, acknowledge your anxieties, insecurities and fears. Write them down: just the simple fact of putting them down on paper and acknowledging them can help you to get a good night's sleep.**

Have a good night!

IRRITABLE BOWEL SYNDROME

Q: *Please can you tell me more about the causes of irritable bowel syndrome, and how it can be treated with complementary medicine?*

A: I see many clients with irritable bowel syndrome (IBS) – indeed it is an all too common complaint nowadays. IBS is also known as spastic colon, or mucous colitis (inflammation of the colon). It is usually characterised by pain, bloating, constipation and diarrhoea, or alternating episodes of each. The causes of IBS include:

- **Chronic constipation**
- **Food allergies: the most common offenders are wheat, corn, milk and dairy products (remember cow's milk is not for everyone), peanuts, fruits (especially citrus), coffee and tea**
- **Too many over-refined and/or fried foods in the diet**
- **Hurried meals and over-drinking alongside meals (It is important to let the body break down food with the hydrochloric acid and enzymes present in the stomach: drinking with a meal dilutes them. Wait 20 minutes before and after a meal to drink.)**
- **Emotional stress, overwork, anxiety, lack of sleep, hurried lifestyle, frustration etc**
- **Overuse of antibiotics**
- **Abuse of laxatives.**

Constipation is a holding on, a tightening of the muscles such that elimination or release cannot take place. People with constipation may be controlling, dominating and find it hard to be spontaneous. Letting go means trusting that life will resolve itself. It means learning how to play and express yourself freely, and how to be at peace with whatever happens.

Diarrhoea can mean that the sufferer has difficulty digesting, and no desire to hold on to anything or any information that is overwhelming or fear-provoking. If you are the type that rushes through life without stopping to listen and absorb what is being said, then the message here is to slow down, take time to listen, and absorb one situation fully before moving on to the next one.

The intestines are where we hold on to those issues that we are afraid to let go of, where our outer reality connects with our inner reality. They indicate how at peace we are with ourselves and the world around us.

To help alleviate IBS, try the following options:

- **Eliminate potential problem foods or drinks from your diet for a week to see if you notice an improvement in your health. It is best to eliminate foods or drinks one at a time to make it easier to identify the ones that may be causing the problem.**
- **Turn detective: keep a diary of your life and bowel habits. Pay special attention to events, stresses or hormonal changes relating to your bowel habits. You may discover the factors that trigger an attack and learn how to prevent future problems.**
- **Graze: instead of eating 3 large meals a day, try eating 5 / 6 smaller meals. Between meals, nuts and seeds (eg almonds, hazelnuts, sunflower seeds etc) are a good option to maintain blood sugar levels, balance the hormones and hence stabilise the mood.**
- **Eat foods rich in fibre such as whole grains and fresh vegetables. Remember that the best time to eat fruit is actually at the beginning of a meal: it can cause indigestion if eaten as a desert. Try psyllium husks, oat bran and ground flax seeds, all of which are available in your local health store.**
- **Avoid sugar, as it can cause fluctuations in blood sugar levels, and also fermentation which can affect the digestion of food.**
- **Drink at least 8 - 10 glasses of filtered water daily.**
- **Keep coffee and tea at a minimum, as they can dehydrate and irritate the colon.**
- **Chill out! Many IBS sufferers appear cool, calm and collected on the surface while holding much anxiety and anticipation inside. This causes tension on the colon. So don't be too uptight: express yourself!**
- **Yoga and meditation are natural tranquillisers that help you physically, emotionally and mentally: so try joining a local class.**
- **Exercise helps to relieve stress and release endorphins, the body's natural painkillers. Exercise also improves muscle tone and bowel tone.**

There are a number of remedies that can help with IBS, including Lycopodium and Nux Vomica. However, in this instance I would strongly recommend a detailed consultation with your local homeopath, as this can help to identify and address any maintaining causes, as well as ensuring you take the right remedy. Finally, it is also important to recognize that if your condition persists, you should consult with a registered health practitioner in case your symptoms indicate other, more serious conditions.

MENOPAUSE

Q: *I wonder if you can help me. I am 59 years old and am suffering from severe hot flushes and sweats and low feelings. I had my womb out 17 years ago and was on HRT for 5 years, but the doctor took me off a few years ago. I would love to wake up in the morning feeling good in myself. Can you recommend anything? I am taking Femillon but I don't feel any different.*

A:Well done for your letter – it takes great courage to write. It is not normal for the body to experience menopausal symptoms on an ongoing basis – your body is trying to tell you that it is out of balance. I have found the following three remedies very effective in helping clients to move forward with courage, confidence and trust, hence improving their quality of life and making their existence more joyful and fun. Match your symptoms to the most suitable remedy picture and take a 30 potency twice daily for two weeks. Then wait and observe for two weeks, before repeating if necessary.

LACHESIS: Sudden heat blushes rising up from the ground. Redness of neck and face. May wake up with a headache. Doesn't like anything tight around the neck or waist. Depression and irritability, tendency to unwarranted suspicion, envy and jealousy. May be excitable, forgetful or hysterical, and behave like a crazy person. Hurry in everything they do and can be very talkative.

PULSATILLA: Hot flushes of the face, and the rest of the body feels chilly. Hot flushes worse indoors and from heat of the bed. They are always pleasing outwardly but are not pleasing themselves enough, and hence become resentful of life. Very weepy, needy and may suffer from depression. Blame everyone for their problems, as they feel unloved and abandoned. Crave sympathy. Moods are changeable. Insomnia worse from 3 to 5 am. Can put on weight easily.

SEPIA: Hot flushes with profuse perspiration. Offensive smelling sweats. Fatigue worse at 5pm, or on waking up at 5 am. Indifferent to loved ones and can be very irritable. Low sex drive. Feel better for exercise or dancing. Depression is more from boredom and despair. Worse on waking, better for being up and moving. Weight gain, especially like a spare tyre around the middle of the body. Bladder can be very weak with involuntary urination on coughing.

Try the following in your diet / lifestyle and see if they help:

- **Drink no more than 2 cups of tea / coffee per day in total, and also drink 8 – 10 glasses of filtered water daily.**
- **Cut out sugar from your diet.**
- **Exercise daily if possible x 20 minutes.**
- **Eat 6 veg / 2 fruit daily.**
- **Cut down / out all dairy (ie milk / cheese). Your calcium is better absorbed in an alkaline body rather than acidic, which dairy creates. If you are worried about lack of calcium in your body, then try a New Era homeopathic tissue salt Cal Phos daily (available at most health shops).**
- **Think positively and affirm to yourself daily that you are well: you are what you think.**

PILES

Q: *I am a 69 year old married lady suffering from piles. My doctor gave me pessaries and an ointment to treat them, but they have not gone away. The practice nurse told me I could have surgery to remove the piles, but I am afraid of hospitals. How serious a condition are piles, and if I have surgery, how long would the procedure take? Also, could you suggest any natural alternatives to surgery?*

A: I do sympathise with you having suffered from piles myself. The good news is they are treatable – however it may take months of natural treatment and years of watching your diet. Haemorrhoids (or piles as they are more commonly known) are varicose veins around the anal canal area. "Varicose" means dilated and swollen. The piles may protrude or remain internal, and they can be very painful. Blood discharges when passing stool is a common symptom.

I don't feel surgery is the answer. Cutting away the piles still doesn't deal with the internal weakness in the portal (or liver) area that may be causing the problem. True healing takes place from the inside out, not from the outside in. Your piles may also be due to a constitutional weakness, especially if you have varicose veins in your legs. Childbirth, diet, lifestyle and hormones can also be factors. In terms of homeopathic remedies, there are several that offer temporary help, but in my experience a constitutional remedy will usually be needed. See if any of the remedies below match your symptoms. Take a 30 potency morning and evening for two weeks, then take a break for two weeks, and then repeat this process monthly for a few months.

SEPIA: Feeling of general collapse in lower organs after giving birth. May crave chocolate. Sepia works on portal circulation, helps to balance hormones, and is an excellent remedy for piles and weak bladder.

LYCOPODIUM: Hard stool, difficult to expel, with blood present. Haemorrhoids very painful to the touch. Lots of wind. Craves sweet foods and products. Sharp shooting pain.

NUX VOMICA: Very painful, itchy piles. Constipation with frequent and ineffectual urging at stool. Unfinished sensation after stool. Insomnia after mental strain, abuse of coffee, alcohol or tobacco.

AESCULUS: Burning piles (piles can protrude and resemble a bunch of grapes). Sharp shooting pain. Apply Aesculus cream.

HAEMAMELIS: Piles are bruised and sore. Bursting feeling, and they continually bleed. Apply Haemamelis cream.

Practical advice for piles is as follows:

- **Take Lepicol (Psyllium husks with acidophyllodus and digestive enzymes), 2 teaspoons in fruit juice each morning. This helps to detoxify the colon and not make it lazy like some other products on the market.**
- **Don't drink water or milk with your food, as this dilutes the digestive enzymes, making it harder to break down food. Drink 20 minutes before or after eating.**
- **Add linseeds or sesame seeds to your cereal.**
- **Continue to eat a high fibre diet, with 6 veg / 2 fruit daily if possible.**
- **Cut out dairy, sugary, refined and processed foods, such as white flour products, milk, cheese etc: these can cause excess mucus in the body, which can contribute to constipation and piles.**
- **Hydrate your body daily with 8 - 10 glasses of filtered water a day (not at mealtimes).**

Haemorrhoids can also relate to a fear of letting go, fear of deadlines, anger from the past, or feeling burdened. So create time and space in your life to enjoy the things you want to do. Create more inner sanctuary time and feel the rewards in your body.

PMT

Q: *I suffer terribly from pre-menstrual tension (PMT). I am very irritable and feel very down coming up to my periods. I snap at my hubby and kids, and I crave lots of chocolate, although I feel worse after eating it. Any advice you could offer would be gratefully received.*

A: Thank you for writing to me about this all too common complaint. Some women are more prone than others to PMT, the mental and emotional tension that arise before the onset of a woman's period, usually due to a slight hormonal imbalance.

PMT often brings up issues to do with how we feel about being a woman, and our relationship to our femininity. It is very hard to be a career woman, a wife, perhaps running a business, running a home and raising children ... and to have a period included on top of all these things! So is there a balance between yourself, your hubby, children, work and home in your life? I'm wondering do you get inner sanctuary time for yourself? Do you discuss issues with your hubby and children, and have a regular family meeting about how you feel about sharing some of your workload? This can help to stop resentment building up. If resentment does build up, then it can lead to anger and – oops! – somebody has to get told off!

So, ask yourself this question next time you feel down and angry: "Am I responsible for my mood?" The answer is Yes! – you own your mood - and remember that your family absorb it too. Also ask yourself "Can I do something about my mood?" Again the answer is Yes! Arrange that family meeting every week and make sure it's ongoing. Exercise more – for example join a Yoga / Pilates class – to help balance your hormones. Cut out chocolate and sugar from your diet (both can greatly affect your mood). And last, but not least, create more inner sanctuary time for yourself, and just yourself, whether it be a relaxing massage, a meditation, or a long bath soaking in aromatherapy essential oils like clary sage or geranium. Go for it and watch yourself become more empowered and at peace with yourself over the coming months – you're worth it!

There are several homeopathic medicines that can alleviate PMT: these include Chamomilla, Lachesis, Mag Phos, Nat Mur, Pulsatilla and Sepia. From what you say, Pulsatilla might be the best remedy for you, as it would help to empower you to make changes in your life, and to cleanse your lymphatic system. However, to choose the remedy which is best suited to your needs, I would recommend you consult with your local homeopath.

SHOCK

Q: *I was involved in a car accident recently. Fortunately I wasn't too badly hurt, but it gave me a real fright. A friend who was on your homeopathic first aid course gave me a remedy, and it really helped me to get over the shock. Can you tell me what the remedy was? – I would like to be prepared for the future!*

A: I'm sorry to hear of your accident, but delighted to learn that the homeopathic remedies helped you! Shock is caused by a sudden fall in the amount of circulating blood, which leads to a lack of oxygen in the tissues and organs, making breathing rapid and shallow. Signs and symptoms of shock include:

- **Weak pulse**
- **Shallow breathing**
- **Cold, pale skin**
- **Fainting and anxiety.**

A degree of shock can occur after an injury, illness or emotional trauma. It can also occur during an infection or allergic reaction. Your friend probably gave you Arnica for the shock (it would also have helped to reduce any bruising). I also use Aconite to treat shock, depending on the circumstances, as outlined below:

ARNICA is a wonderful remedy for shock following an accident, and also helps with bruising. In emergencies, repeat the 30 potency every 30 minutes. As mentioned elsewhere in this book, always assess any injury before using Arnica, as it may mask a fracture by reducing the pain and swelling.

ACONITE is an excellent remedy to treat the panic that can set in following shocks. It is also a really effective remedy for terror, fear of death or ailments from fright. Aconite can also be used to help a person recover from a past event or experience that has left them with deep physical or emotional scars.

For future reference, you can also try the following flower remedies for shock:

- **Star of Bethlehem** for all types of shock, including the shock of giving birth
- **Bach Flower Rescue Remedy**
- **Emergency Essence from Jan de Vries**, a blend of essences of chamomile, lavender, red clover, purple cornflower, selfheal and yarrow: this has a gentle, calming and rebalancing action.

If you are suffering from the aftermath of a shock, you may also find it useful to talk about the accident, rather than bottling up your feelings. If you find yourself unable or unwilling to talk to close friends and family, then counselling might be a good option.

I'm glad that you weren't badly injured in the accident. However, and on a more general note, if shock follows a severe accident, remember that you should seek medical help immediately! Keep the person warm, and loosen any tight clothing. Do not move the person if they are unconscious or have a serious injury. Otherwise move the head to a position lower than the body so that the blood drains back to the head.

SUNBURN & SUNSTROKE

Q: *We are off on our holidays soon to Turkey. Please can you give me any tips or recommend any homeopathic remedies to use in case any of our children get sunburn?*

A: Sunburn is a very unpleasant condition. Babies and children are particularly vulnerable as their skin is thinner and more sensitive than adult skin. Prevention is the best way to avoid sunburn and its unpleasant consequences. It is highly advisable to use sun creams with a high sun protection factor (SPF), and total block for babies and younger children. Non-allergic, good quality sun creams are available from all good chemists.

Sunstroke occurs when a person gets overheated from too much exposure to the sun in very hot weather, or from too much exertion in the heat. Signs and symptoms of sunstroke include high fever, inability to perspire, red hot skin, headache, nausea and a fast pulse.

In extreme cases, a person may lose consciousness. Sunstroke can be serious, and may need urgent medical attention, especially in younger children. The following remedies can help with sunburn and sunstroke:

BELLADONNA: High fever. Hot, red, burning skin. Throbbing headache. Child may become delirious and have dilated pupils. Use a 30 potency half hourly until symptoms are relieved. Belladonna is the best remedy for sunburn and sunstroke.

APIS: Use if the skin becomes swollen and puffy after exposure to the sun. Stinging and burning pains. Fever. Use a 30 potency hourly until symptoms are relieved.

Practical advice for sunburn and sunstroke is as follows:

- **Cover up, protect with cream, and don't over-exposure yourself**
- **Babies under one year old should not be exposed to the sun at all**
- **Allow short periods of exposure to the sun so that you can acclimatise to it**

- **Tropical treatments like Aloe Vera and cucumber slices can be soothing on sunburn**
- **Ensure that you are hydrated, as dehydration can lead to headaches and even sunstroke**
- **If you suspect sunstroke, move the person to a shady area out of the sun, cool them down with tepid water and plenty of fluids (not alcohol), and seek medical advice.**

Happy holidays!

THORNS

Q: *After a recent spot of gardening, I ended up with a tiny thorn in my finger. Try as I might, I can't remove it. A friend told me there is a homeopathic remedy that can help: which is it?*

A: Your friend is right! The homeopathic remedy Silicea can help to remove deeply embedded thorns. This is another of those remedies that seems to have a magical effect. It is particularly useful if you have a painful thorn or splinter which cannot be removed because it is so deeply embedded, or because it has no head. Use a 30 potency 4 to 8 hourly and watch the thorn dislodge itself before your very eyes! You can also use Silicea after the removal of a tooth to help the body eject any bone splinters.

I have a friend who was very sceptical about homeopathy until she successfully used Silicea to remove a thorn which had been embedded in her finger for weeks. The thorn had resisted all attempts to remove it until she tried this wonderfully effective remedy!

5
EMOTIONAL WELL-BEING

ANXIETY

At some stage in our lives, all of us experience anxiety: about money and bills, exams, exam results, job interviews, bird 'flu and so on. Anxiety is where we worry about possible negative outcomes rather than maintaining an attitude of optimism and trust in our own capacity to cope with whatever comes our way. We fear not something concrete, but something that ***might*** happen. In this way anxiety limits us, and means we dare not take risks. Our lives can become terribly constrained by this fear of what may or may not happen.

Sometimes this attitude is engendered by our parents always telling us not to do things for fear of what might happen to us. This habit of fastening attention on to the negative can become a way of life. Worse still, negative intention can create negative experience. Negative emotions sap energy, whereas joy and laughter nurture us.

Anxiety is endemic in contemporary society. Our emotional antennae are primed to respond to the pace of life with panic. Living, as most of us do, under tremendous stress, we become easy prey. Anxiety about health can become a major obsession, with concern over symptoms often masking the real anxiety – a fear of death. In this instance, many people expend a lot of energy and effort searching for medicinal answers rather than trying to address the cause of their neurotic anxiety. In the 1950's, drug addiction was created by prescribing tranquillisers like Valium for years on end. But Valium didn't solve anxiety – all it did was to suppress the problem. The 1980's saw the rise of the "Prozac Generation", where people preferred – or were advised - to take anti-depressants to take the edge off their feelings (both positive and negative), rather than making changes in their life or finding better ways of dealing with their problems and anxieties.

There are several homeopathic remedies which can help with anxiety. Choose the remedy which most closely matches the symptoms, and take a 30 potency every morning and evening for no longer than two weeks. If your symptoms start to improve sooner, then stop taking the remedies.

ARSENICUM: Person may be obsessive about tidiness, and have constant worries, especially about their health. They often have many tests done which reveal nothing pathological, ie nothing physically wrong. This reassures them temporarily, but the anxiety soon returns and once again they become hypochondriacal.

ARGENTUM NITRICUM: Good for obsessive disorders, panic attacks, claustrophobia and agoraphobia. Person is easily overwhelmed by feelings of panic, becoming restless and agitated. They find it impossible to stop their minds from running over improbable disaster scenarios.

RHUS TOX: Useful for people with superstitious behavioural patterns, eg not stepping on the cracks in pavements, or compulsively checking that everything electrical is turned off in the house and that the back door is locked.

SILICEA: Good for people who feel shy and unconfident, and who withdraw into their own private world whenever they feel exposed in public settings.

When I treat people suffering from anxiety, I tell them they have the following lesson to learn:

Try letting go of the need to be too controlling in your life. Trust more, and go with the synchronicity and flow of life. Embrace change at all times: otherwise the energy in your body stays stagnant and may lead to a fear that something bad might happen. Keep working on removing the old, negative thought patterns, and affirm to yourself daily:

"I trust. Thy will be done."

Let the higher source of energy – be it the universal energy, or God – take away your problems to be solved.

EXAM HEADACHES

Q: *My fifteen year old daughter is currently studying hard for her exams, but has started to suffer from tension headaches. They usually come on in the afternoon, and her energy always seems to be low in the early afternoon. She is a perfectionist who compares herself to everyone else. If she gets 90% in an exam, she will say "where did I go wrong?" She is quite sporty, but sometimes has a short temper. She has been to see a consultant about the headaches, and he has put her on Amitryptaline. Are there any natural homeopathic remedies that could help her?*

A: Thanks for your question. I know that it is not easy to be a parent during the stress-filled time of exams – all you can do at the moment is just to be there and support your daughter. From what you describe, she may be suffering from electromagnetic stress, brought on by an overactive mind. This means that her energy is stuck in her head area - all the headaches are doing is trying to release this excess, pent-up energy in this area. In many of my clients, I often see high energy in the head area and low physical energy in the rest of the body.

Encourage your daughter to stop comparing herself to other people. She is unique and has to see all the positives in her life: this means focussing on the 90% scored in her exam and not the 10% lost! She has to understand that she is trying to do her best at all times, and that her best is good enough. You can reassure her in this respect.

If she has a mobile phone, she needs to protect herself against potentially harmful radiation with a magnetic waveshield. Make sure that there is nothing electrical within 3 feet of where she is sleeping. Some people are very susceptible to the electromagnetic stress caused by electrical items like mobiles, TV's, PC's, pylons etc, and this stress can lead to headaches. Encourage her to keep doing sport, as fresh air and exercise both help to balance the energy in the body and head. Promote a healthy diet for her, including things like chicken, fish, salads, fruit, vegetables and so on. Cut out sugars from her diet. She can also try one of the following remedies. Match her symptoms to the most suitable remedy picture and take a 30 potency twice daily for two weeks. Then wait and observe for two weeks, before repeating if necessary. Nux Vomica aids concentration and focus, whilst Aurum brings more joy and love into the heart, and relieves the perceived burden of responsibility.

NUX VOMICA: Irritable, impatient, ambitious, competitive and driven. May be a workaholic. Easily offended and can lose temper easily: anger at contradiction from others. Possible insomnia from worry about exams or deadlines. Tendency to break things from anger and frustration. Energy worse around 2 pm. Fastidious, can become especially angry if objects are not in their proper place. Their minds think very fast and can leap from one idea to the next.

AURUM: Perfectionist, always going for gold. Very intense, ambitious and idealistic: they set very high goals for themselves and fear failure and heights. Outbursts of anger and extreme irritability. May wake up 3 - 4 hours after falling asleep. Severe, chronic insomnia. May feel low and depressed.

I would also suggest trying a bush flower essence called "Calm & Clear." Rosemary aromatherapy essential oil is also very useful and aids study. Place a few drops on a tissue nearby and do the same on the day of the exams. This oil aids memory and encourages the olfactory area of the brain to remember what you studied previously.

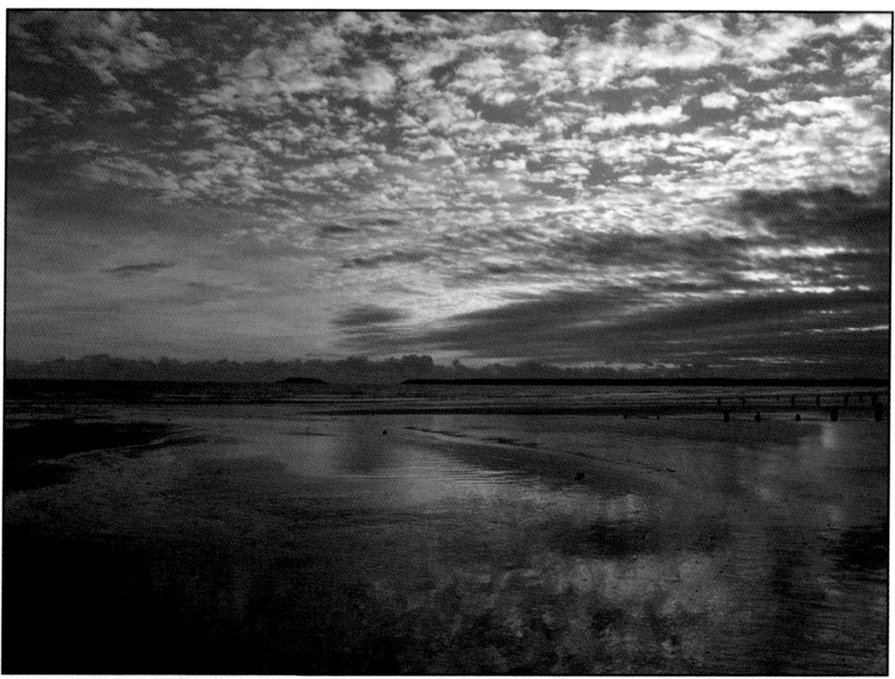

"Freedom of the mind is the greatest form of freedom."

HEALING HURTS – PART 1

We have all been hurt at some stage in our lives: failed romances, broken promises, a let-down in our personal lives, the loss of a loved one or a favourite pet, or missing out on a hoped-for promotion at work. Feeling hurt like this can lead to sadness, tears, anxiety in the stomach, loss of appetite and so on. The feeling of being hurt is a natural experience: it is something we all go through, and something we must all deal with. But if we suppress our true, core values, if we avoid facing up to our current circumstances, and if we allow those feelings of hurt to continue unchecked, then we run the risk of allowing those feelings to impact negatively on our lives – and worse, to potentially undermine our own health and well-being.

People react differently to being hurt. It can knock their confidence and self-esteem, and lead to anger being stored in their liver or heart. Others may choose to put up a wall to isolate themselves, hide their true feelings, and - for example - may decide not to enter into another relationship for fear of being hurt again.

When we hold on to hurt feelings for too long, we continue to punish ourselves – we feel that we are bad and deserve to be punished. Guilt is often present as a way of not taking responsibility. But guilt is an emotion to warn us that we are doing something inconsistent with our true values. So when we feel guilt, we need to reassess our values, forgive the past behaviour which helped us to learn – and make changes in our lives. Remember: guilt is sometimes called "resentment turned inwards."

There are five positive steps we can take to help heal the hurt:

(1) Identify the feeling. Do you feel used, abandoned, angry, resentful, misunderstood or hurt?

(2) Sense the first time this was triggered in childhood.

(3) If your hurt was caused by another person, forgive them, even if they were in the wrong. Send love and light to the person that you feel has let you down. By doing this you release your anger. Anger is a very negative emotion which can lead to many health problems, such as arthritis, high blood pressure and

sinusitis to name but a few. So open up your heart and try to heal the situation.

(4) Visualise yourself responding in a different way.

(5) Do it!

From experience, I know that many of my clients find it difficult to forgive and move on. This is why I use homeopathic medicines and flower essences to help make the transition easier. The healing process can be a long and tough journey, but it is made much easier once you have taken that first step!

HEALING HURTS – PART 2

Holding on to hurt can have negative consequences for our health and well-being. When your body is holding on to a hurt feeling, then you can feel sadness, anger or regret. I encourage my clients to let go of issues that happened in the past, to live fully in the present, and to hand over situations that are out of their control to a higher level. I give the following affirmation for letting go and trusting that everything will be resolved in the end:

"I am willing to surrender this situation to my creator right now, and when I do, everything turns out perfectly."

This affirmation helps my clients to stop worrying and creates a more positive outlook. Say it three times every morning and evening until no longer needed, and then say, "It is done." Also try sending love and light to the person that has done you an injustice. By doing this you heal your own energies and dissolve the sadness and anger residing in your body.

The following homeopathic remedies can also help to release anger and make sad cells happier:

NAT MUR: Person feels let down, disappointed or betrayed. Fear of being emotionally hurt in the future, so becomes reserved and unapproachable. Keeps their feelings to themselves. Will only cry when alone (silent grief) or cannot cry at all. Dwells on past, disagreeable occurrences. Feels very angry and vengeful. May have a history of big problems or quarrels with parents. Desires salt. Hates being consoled. Hatred of person who has offended them.

IGNATIA: Feels tremendous grief at the end of a relationship. Grief with insomnia. Sighs a lot. Inability to swallow because of the sensation of a lump in the throat (this is associated with unexpressed tears). Sense of hopelessness is created from being hurt or disappointed.

AURUM: Suicidal feelings develop after a prolonged period of grieving. Person suffers deep feelings of despair and does not want to live.

LEAVING CERT BLUES

Q: *I have just finished my leaving cert exams. I feel I may not have done as well as I would have liked. I now live in fear of failing them and am afraid of the outcome. Are there any homeopathic remedies that could help me to relax and stop worrying?*

A: My heart goes out to all students who have just completed their leaving cert and who are awaiting their results. The period between exams and results is a time of great indecision and fear of the future. Your letter took me back to my own memories of my leaving cert. I too felt unsure at the time of what path to take, and was really fearful about my results.

But really, you now have to trust that the outcome will be OK. Stop worrying and hand over your fears. My feeling is that whatever results you get in the points system will be suitable for what you may do for the future. Stop being too hard on yourself. Whatever you decide to do for the future, be sure that you are passionate about it. In other words, decide intuitively from within how you feel about the path you take. Do not choose a direction simply because that is what your parents want you to do. Do it for yourself and not to please anyone else. I see too many people in my clinics who wish that they had listened to their own inner guidance rather than listening to their head and operating out of fear.

The following remedy may help put an end to your jitteriness and worries from anticipation. It should also help you to feel more relaxed.

LYCOPODIUM: Person fears the future too much, has a fear of losing control, and craves sweet things. Has a negative outlook and is lacking in confidence and self-esteem.

Please try and trust that everything will be OK, and keep saying the following positive affirmation to yourself morning and evening:

"Everything is in divine and perfect order right now."

Good luck. I wish you every success in your future. Simply by being positive, the outcome is always better.

LOSS & GRIEF

Many of us become emotionally crippled through the experience of a loss. Not just the loss of a loved one – but also the loss of a pet, a job or a house, or a child leaving home for university. You may experience loss as abandonment. The loss of a relationship may feel like a mini-death: you may feel shocked, wounded or betrayed if the person you have been involved with leaves of their own volition. You may no longer feel connected to the world through the one you love, and you may also feel isolated and alone. Sometimes we are crippled because we let these feelings take over in our lives, and we withdraw into a cocoon.

Grief and loss can produce an armouring around your heart which initially seems protective, but which does not really protect you at all. In fact this armour usually prevents you from feeling any kind of love, and your heart becomes hardened to the possibility of opening up again. Author Stephen Levine describes grief as "unfinished business." He says we often feel a sense of loss due to the awareness that we could have had so much more with a person. We regret that we could not fully allow that person to get close, or that we needed more. This increases the sense of separation and ultimate aloneness. A feeling of emptiness makes you hang on to regrets about the past, and become stuck with longing for more, even though the other person is no longer there.

The challenge of loss is to try and trust in the greater wisdom of the universe, for we cannot always understand why we are forced to let go of people and situations we love, and to move on. If we can find the courage to let go, then we can experience the pleasures of making new connections, building new relationships and opening up to love again. I have focussed here on the loss of a relationship: but the lessons to be learnt apply equally to the other sorts of loss we all face throughout our lives.

Coming to terms with loss involves resolving to live more fully in each and every moment, rather than hanging on to the incomplete past or shielding yourself against the present. I was fortunate enough to have a wise old grand-aunt, Hanora, and she taught me the following poem:

"If memories of days gone by
Are darkened by regrets and sorrow,
Just look ahead and build
Sweet memories for tomorrow."

Turn a negative into a positive, and be more optimistic for the future.

PANIC ATTACKS

Q: *I suffer from panic attacks. My heart races and I feel as if I am going to die. As a result of the attacks, I have become housebound. Could homeopathy help me?*

A: Yes, homeopathy can help you. Panic attacks typically occur because of a shock or fright to the body. The shock or fright is maintained within the body's cells, and can manifest itself - sometimes years later - in many different ways, for example as palpitations, tightness in the throat or chest area, difficulties in swallowing, a sensation of butterflies in the stomach, or, as in your case, becoming housebound.

In homeopathy, we always look for the reason behind the patient's symptoms: there are remedies that can help you to overcome the symptoms, but it is also crucial to identify what is causing the problem. There are many potential reasons for panic attacks. It may be that you have never been well since a frightful experience, for example a car accident, the loss of a family member, being stuck in a lift, or witnessing an accident or trauma. Or the cause might be something unknown to you, a trauma that occurred too far back in the past for you to consciously remember it. The following remedy should help you: take a 30 potency twice daily for one to two weeks, until the symptoms alleviate.

ACONITE: State of fear and anxiety. Physical and mental restlessness. Person fears death and may feel they are going to die when having a panic attack. Fear of crowds, the future and enclosed spaces. Undertakes many tasks but perseveres in none. Pains may be intolerable and drive the person crazy. Person feels as though the pains come from their stomach, ie butterfly sensation.

If your symptoms do not improve, I suggest you seek further help with your local health practitioner to outrule any other potential maintaining causes for the way you feel.

STRESS

Q: *I run my own business, and am extremely busy at the moment. I work long days and most weekends, and often have to skip lunch. My wife tells me I should delegate more, but I do not trust my staff to do the work to my high standards. I find I now have lots of muscular aches and pains, and generally feel tired all the time. I also keep losing my temper easily. I have started to wake up at 2 o'clock every morning and then find it difficult to get back to sleep. Can you suggest something to help my mind switch off?*

A: You appear to be very stressed out with your business. The homeopathic remedy described below will help, but remember it is crucial to keep a healthy balance between family, work, recreation and time-out. Diet is also important. You should exercise at least twice a week, and eat every four hours in order to avoid low blood-sugar which can interfere with your mood. Avoid excess sugar, coffee and tea, as these can all put a strain on your adrenal glands which are there to help you in times of stress. For a between meals snack, almonds, hazelnuts and sunflower seeds are all good sources of protein. Make sure your diet includes plenty of fresh fruit and vegetables.

Have you ever tried meditation? If you meditate regularly, you will find that with a quieter, more focussed and less cluttered mind, you will be able to make better decisions about both your work and your own life.

Also try the remedy Nux Vomica 30 twice daily for two weeks. This remedy is useful in cases where when the mind finds it difficult to switch off. It also helps to reduce irritability, especially when you find yourself getting angry and impatient. Nux Vomica is often prescribed to people who have the following characteristics:

- **Fastidious about their work**
- **Anxiety is worse in the morning**
- **May crave alcohol, cigarettes or spicy food, but may be worse for all of these.**

Nux Vomica allows you to be fully present in the now, to enjoy the moment, not to worry about the past and to look forward to the future. Good luck!

An additional note: in homeopathy, one single remedy is often used to treat a number of ailments. Nux Vomica is a case in point. It is the number one remedy for treating a hangover, and is also used for indigestion, heartburn, nausea, retching and vomiting.

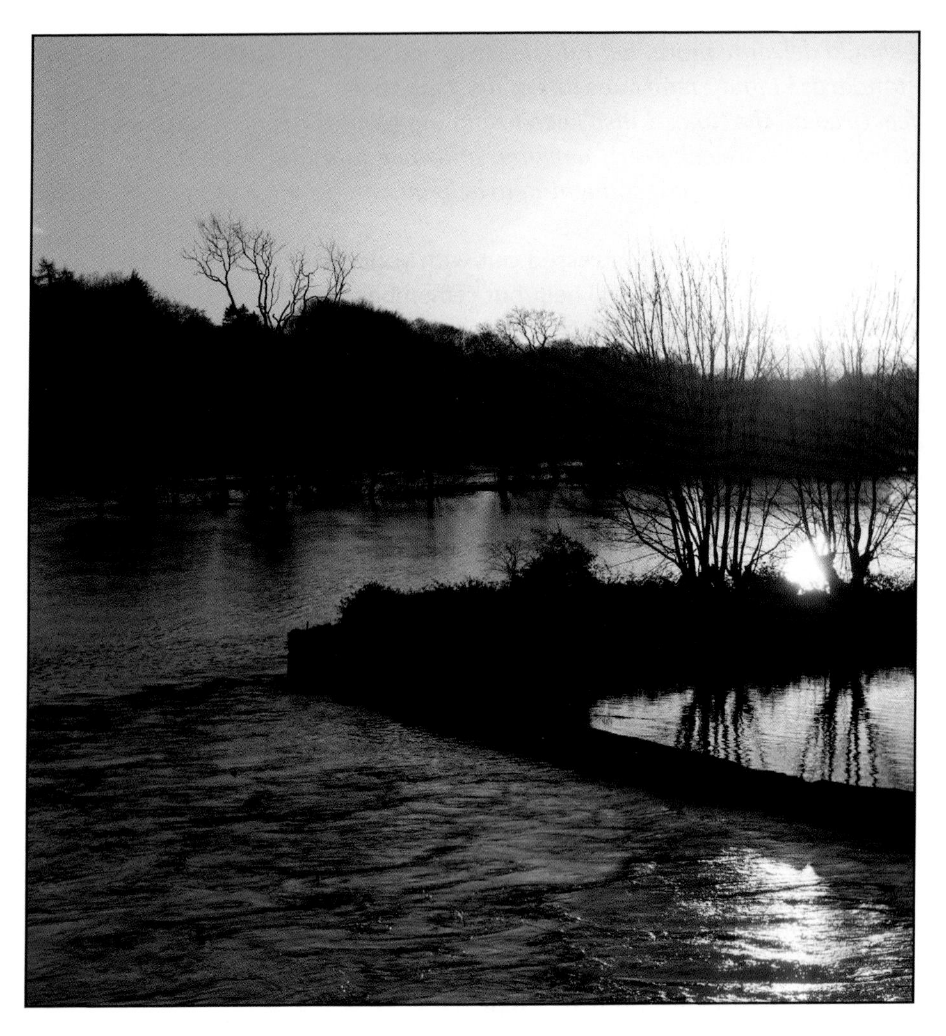

"Live every day that dawns as if it is your last."

SUICIDE IS NOT THE ANSWER – SO WHAT IS? PART 1

I must admit I thought long and hard before about writing about suicide, as it is such a difficult and sensitive issue. But for any family that has been touched by suicide, I hope that this article can provide some words of comfort and healing. And I also hope that the other articles on this topic can provide some hope and inspiration for people who are feeling depressed, by looking at some of the things that need to be done, both by themselves and by society at large.

We are seemingly surrounded by an epidemic of suicides at the moment. My heart goes out to anyone who has suffered a bereavement in these tragic circumstances. In many cases, family and friends had no idea that the person was feeling so depressed. "If only they'd talked to me," they say, or "He was the last person I would have thought would do that." But what is it that makes people feel so low that it makes them consider ending their lives? Where does the pain come from?

In my clinics, I have seen a number of individuals who live on the edge. They feel they cannot endure the pain of living, and often turn to alcohol or drugs to numb the pain. However, once the effect of the alcohol or drugs has worn off, the pain keeps returning. And it will keep on returning until it is acknowledged and healed. Not everyone turns to alcohol and drugs, however. Some people hide their feelings and become introverted. They put a wall around themselves, in the vain hope that if they don't talk about it and if nobody knows about it, then the pain might go away. But the wall only prevents further hurts – it does nothing to address the underlying pain, and may make people even more sensitive to the blocked emotions inside. This can lead to them making false assumptions in their minds, and taking everything far too personally.

Other people may have extreme feelings of anger which they cannot express, and which they suppress. The result of this anger turned inwards is depression. But it is not just unexpressed anger that can go inwards. Unexpressed grief can also stir up energy in us that needs to be discharged. If it is not released, it can lead to chronic depression, shock, anxiety, nervousness, resentment, sadness, confusion, guilt, shame, or indeed a numbness – no feeling at all. Physical conditions like sleeplessness, aches, skin diseases and so on can also develop.

The pains that people suffer from may be summarised as follows:

- **A loss or great disappointment in their lives.**
- **A loss of love for themselves, hence making them feel abandoned and lost – "I am not worthy."**
- **A feeling that they cannot live in the supposedly perfect real world: they compare themselves too much to others, don't accept themselves as they are, and hence feel they are not worthy to be living, and that the world would be a better place without them.**

Clearly, if someone feels suicidal, they are greatly out of balance. Yet we are all born into this world in a simple, pure, blissful state, full of love. You only have to look at a newborn baby to make your heart melt. At the base level, the essence of life is pure love. This pure love never disappears – it just gets hidden away and covered up by the many layers of fear, anger, resentment and sadness. To comprehend our feelings, we need also to comprehend the many layers that we have to work through. When we understand all of our feelings – good and bad – and love ourselves more, we come to know that we are all worthy. Then life suddenly becomes a happier existence and we sail through our life lessons with love instead of fear.

In the next article, I will say more on what can be done both by people who are feeling depressed, and by society as a whole.

SUICIDE IS NOT THE ANSWER – SO WHAT IS? PART 2

In the first part of this article, I wrote about the wave of suicides that seems to be sweeping across the country. So what can be done to help prevent further outbreaks? There are internal and external factors at play here – both at an individual level and from the point of view of society.

One of the first steps is to acknowledge that we all have two basic types of feelings or emotions: joyful and painful. Both are necessary parts of our very existence, and help us to grow and learn throughout our lives. When we are full of joy, we feel strong, happy and fulfilled. When we are full of pain, we feel weak, depleted and alone. But painful emotions often serve a purpose and point us towards an area in our lives that needs attention. If you are full of painful feelings, you need to talk about them with safe and supportive people.

My instincts tell me that there needs to be a sea change in attitudes across the country. I believe governments should add a new lesson to the school curriculum, covering "Awareness of self and life." Our kids learn English, Science and Maths, so why not teach them from the age of seven on how to interpret their feelings and emotions? This should be seen as a normal subject for everyone to study. I realise that teaching children about such "life lessons" may seem an extreme measure, but if we are serious about addressing the issue of suicide, then we need to do something – prevention is better when "cure" is not an option. It is not sufficient to have counsellors on a part time basis. Students at secondary school level will simply be too embarrassed or too shy to admit they have a problem. If we start early with educating our children, the ripple effect of their awareness and healing can grow outwardly to their parents, and indeed on to their own children as time goes by.

Some people have lost touch with the simple things in life, such as a walk in nature, a love for animals, or just being still and admiring the beauty of a rainbow or a sunset. Why is this important? Because if small things like this can give you pleasure, then you may not be so depressed about lacking the latest gadgets that seem to be taking over our lives. Too many people live their lives in the fast lane, where their heads are constantly bombarded with unwanted thoughts that never seem to stop. Why not teach children how to quieten the mind and to listen to their own intuition? Believe it or not, each of us typically has between 60,000 – 90,000 thoughts a day. This is not a problem if those thoughts are positive – but if they are negative, they can be destructive. Our overactive minds are not helped by the over-use of mobile phones, computers, playstations and so on causing electromagnetic stress. If you are feeling depressed, you need to focus on what you do have – not on what you don't have.

As a society, we also need to change the way we think about depression, mental illness and suicide. I met a guy recently who told me he shared a house with several other guys. He was suffering from depression, but none of his friends or flatmates knew, because he was afraid of what their reaction would be. This kind of stigma and attitude needs to be demolished. In this respect, it is very constructive when well-known personalities are open about their own bouts of depression and suicidal thoughts – anyone, from any walk of life, can be prone to such thoughts, but they can be overcome. As the saying goes, "the night is always darkest just before dawn."

We are taught religion at school, but I believe that in order to worship outwardly, we also need to worship inwardly first. There is a God inside each and every individual. The best way to show love is to give love and be open to receiving it. If you love yourself enough, then love is shared unconditionally to all mankind. When self-awareness and healing of our own physical, mental, emotional and spiritual body become automatic, only then I believe will we have fewer suicides.

SUICIDE IS NOT THE ANSWER – SO WHAT IS? PART 3

Q: *Sometimes I get suicidal. I feel a build up of anger in me, and my head starts to spin. It is in this state that I have taken myself to the edge to end it all. Could you give me any advice or suggestions that I could carry around with me to read whenever I feel like this, to help me deal with the state I get into. I am seeing a psychiatrist and am getting counselling at the moment, but can you offer any help too?*

A:Thank you for your honest and heart-rending question. It must have taken a lot of courage for you to write this letter. I have thought long and hard about your question, and the advice here is to guide you to help yourself.

The first key point is for you to observe your thoughts carefully. Try to imagine a separate, objective part of you looking back in at yourself. Feel the anger when it is fermenting, ie before it becomes self-destructive, and try to nip it in the bud. Take five deep breaths, and say to yourself "I acknowledge my anger, but I release it and let it go."

If you feed your negative thoughts, then they can become obsessive and stay stuck. By that I mean the self-destructive thoughts can become like a treadmill – always spinning, and with no gaps in between. On this treadmill, you are connected to pure pain in the body and mind - and your body stores this pain in the negative emotions of anger, sadness, grief, loss, revenge or self-hatred. When you are in this state, you need to get the excess energy out of your head and back into the body (static shocks are often a sign of stressed people who live too much in the head and who need grounding).

The following techniques can also help you to release the excess energy in your head:

Be honest with yourself: the fact that you wrote this letter already says that you are an honest person. Try writing down your destructive thoughts and how you feel about them - the simple fact of identifying and acknowledging these thought patterns will help to weaken their power. Then affirm positively to yourself either silently or out loud "I love me. I am worthy of living." All it takes is 15 seconds of positive thoughts to change the energy in your body.

Talk about / share your feelings: talk to someone about how you feel. If you don't have a close friend or confidant, try the Samaritans, or make sure that you are totally honest with your counsellor or psychiatrist.

Stay fully present in the now: stop your thoughts from going back to the past or going into the unknown of the future. The past may be related to pain, but you cannot change the past. Simply accept it as part of your life's journey. When you stay positive in the present and think positive thoughts daily, then you can expect positive things to happen. Your reward will be inner peace and less negative mental chatter, plus you will automatically become more positive in yourself.

Write down your joy list: write down three positive things you like about yourself and affirm them daily, for example "I love my eyes, I love my hands, I love the way I play guitar." It is vital that you affirm these positive things EVERY DAY! Self love comes first before you can accept other people's love into your life. Your joy list dissolves your self-criticism and self-hatred. Also, have a happy image or place in your mind that you can come back to you in times of need. Focus on what you have rather than what you don't have.

Still the mind passively: when you find yourself thinking destructive thoughts, force yourself to sit quietly and just acknowledge them. If your thoughts are negative, then they do not serve you. So imagine them as a file on your computer – cut and paste the file into your recycle bin, and then press the delete button to empty it. Breathing can also help to still the mind. Focus on your breathing. Slowly breathe in peace, joy and happiness. As you breathe out, just smile to yourself. Practice this five to ten minutes daily and the energy in your body will become more positive.

Let off steam: if you find your head is buzzing constantly and you just cannot be still, then you need to let off steam in a constructive way. Try punching a boxing bag or cushion, exercise until you sweat, or simply scream and yell as loud as you can (make sure you find a suitable place to do this!). All these actions will help you to let go of the negative emotions that need balancing. Exercise of any sort is extremely beneficial in balancing excess energy in the head and putting it back into the body where it belongs.

Take responsibility for where you are at: you may not be the cause of the problem, but you are the only one who can resolve it. And never forget: you are always worth it!

I suffered from depression myself in my twenties, and am only too aware of the darkness. I used positive affirmations and a joy list to help me overcome my depression, and I continue to use them to this day. So it is important to use the above techniques ALL THE TIME whether you are feeling positive or negative: this will help not only to build up your positive energy, but also it will make it easier to overcome negative thoughts when they arise. A final point: research has shown that homeopathic remedies can also help over the longer term to shift your mind patterns to be more positive: consult with your local homeopath.

THE BOOK THAT CHANGED MY LIFE

Many books are written on health, healing and harmony. But there is truly one book for me that started me on my own healing journey – and I can say that it changed my life and helped me to become more aware of myself in a positive way.

In my early 20's, I suffered from depression and was prescribed antidepressants. They altered the chemical balance in my brain, which was therapeutic. But I wanted to know what had caused the chemical imbalance in the first place. I found out that the medication I was on was quite strong and had a number of unpleasant side-effects. At the time, I felt nobody understood the way I felt – not my family, my GP, my friends, my psychiatrist, and least of all myself. I still felt like I had a weak physical body with an overactive mind. This kept bringing out unwelcome symptoms like insomnia, persistent and unwanted thoughts, and wanting to just hide away from the world. I felt so lost and that nobody had the answer. That was until one day when I found a book written by Dr Wayne Dyer called "Your Erroneous Zones." I read this book and it gave me hope, inspiration and the answers I was looking for as to why the body and mind can go so out of balance.

I practiced the positive affirmations and advice given in the book. My thoughts became more positive and hence the physical energy in my body improved too. I vowed to myself that I would do everything in my whole being to learn as much as possible, to never allow myself to go back there to that "Darkness." I spent the following 15 years in London working as a nurse, at the same time as learning about the many natural therapies and techniques that could help me to heal not just myself but also other people on their journey through life.

A thought is energy. If it is positive, it raises your own physical energy. If it is negative, it brings your energy down and leads to fatigue, apathy, lack of motivation and unhappiness. So I thank God for finding me this book, and for all the other inspirational writers like Wayne Dyer. My life is now so full of purpose that I thank my illness for changing my life. For every negative thought there is always a positive. There are many healing, positive books out there that can change your life. I found one, so can you!

Negative emotions block your energy and your purpose here on earth. Positive emotions bring in more joy. Joy is a natural emotion and is freely available to all of us. Remember, there are joyful people living in poverty as well as unhappy people living with great wealth. When you really appreciate what you have got – and not what you haven't got! - all fears dissipate and joy comes to the surface. So say yes to life and no to negative emotions and thoughts.

6
HOMEOPATHY

HOMEOPATHY: A SYMPATHETIC WAY OF HEALING

Q: *I have always been a strong believer in the effectiveness of homeopathy, but as a homeopath, how do you respond to the frequent negative media coverage of this complementary therapy?*

A: You are right, homeopathy often does seem to get more than its fair share of bad press, so thank you for offering me the opportunity to be more positive and enlighten you once more on homeopathy and how it helps people to heal themselves!

I should stress from the start that it is not my intention to criticise conventional medicine. It has been - and continues to be - wonderfully successful in many areas. But it doesn't have all the answers. Conventional medicine most definitely has its place – but so does complementary medicine in general and homeopathy in particular.

Homeopathy is one of the most gentle forms of medicine. It is not about suppressing symptoms and prescribing ever stronger drugs to combat disease: rather it works by stimulating the body's own healing mechanisms and energies, helping the patient to heal themselves. Homeopathy is safe and non-toxic, and can be used alongside conventional therapies.

Homeopathy considers all aspects of a person's being, respecting the fact that everyone is unique and individual. It often acts deeply on the patient, and can have lasting effects on all levels, balancing, as it does, not just the physical, but also the mental, emotional and spiritual aspects of the person. In other words, it takes a holistic approach, treating the whole person and not just the disease.

Homeopathy works on the individual's vital force or energy. Too many people today suffer from fatigue, both physical and mental, and such fatigue can be the first sign that the body is out of balance. Homeopathy helps to rekindle the body's own energy to help it heal itself. If ailments are treated in isolation, and if the patient's whole range of symptoms are not treated together, then the root cause of imbalance is seldom found. Symptoms may disappear, but the disease may merely be suppressed and flare up again as another ailment elsewhere in the body.

Conventional medicine successfully eases the discomfort of many ailments with painkillers, anti-inflammatory drugs and anti-depressants. But as many conventional health practitioners readily recognise themselves, such drugs may not offer a long-term solution. They can have unpleasant side effects, may lead to addiction, and all too often a complete cure remains out of reach.

From my experience of over 15 years in nursing and 20 years in complementary medicine, I believe that disease and illness are not just about viruses, bacteria, parasites, hormonal imbalances, toxins, genetic tendencies, dysfunctional cells and so on. Yes, all these things can and do make a person ill, but there are 1001 other potential factors that can have a major influence on a person's health. These include diet and lifestyle, stress levels at work, geopathic or electromagnetic stress, food allergies, negative thoughts, mercury and metal toxicity, and major life events such as divorce, bereavement and disappointments in love, work, study and so on. Unless all the influences on a person's health are considered together, we as health practitioners may miss the underlying cause of the illness – or imbalance – in the person's body. By focusing on one single element, we run the risk of offering a temporary cure, no cure at all, or worse still, exacerbating the original condition.

I believe that disease is often present to let us know that a person's physical, mental, emotional and spiritual sides need to be treated. As an example, stomach ailments like gastritis or heartburn may be brought on by the person not being able to "stomach" what is going on around them. Or perhaps the heart and lungs are suffering as a result of someone suffering from a letdown, sadness from a loss, or from holding on to anger: and as a result, a physical symptom such as angina or repeated chest infections comes out in the body. If you don't believe about the link between illness and a person's overall well-being, ask someone who suffers from cold sores: often this condition will be at its worst when they are at their lowest ebb, stressed at work, or have suffered from some trauma. By working holistically, homeopathy can help to remove both the blockage and the cause of the blockage (or illness), restoring the person's energy or life-force, and helping them to move on.

Many conventional health practitioners argue that there is no scientific proof that homeopathy works. Whilst this is the case, there is also no scientific proof that it ***doesn't*** work! In its rush to scientifically disprove complementary therapies, conventional medicine conveniently forgets the failings of its beloved science: how long it took to prove a link between smoking and lung cancer, or how thalidomide caused birth defects, or how many so called wonder-drugs have subsequently to be withdrawn when their toxic side-effects are fully understood.

In the end, I can no more prove that homeopathy works than I can prove that the sun will rise tomorrow! My instinct is that it works on levels – or energies – that science does not yet understand. In the absence of "scientific" evidence, surely the best proof that homeopathy does work is shown by the huge numbers of people – including myself, my family, friends and clients - across the world who have experienced firsthand the benefits of homeopathy and seen how effective this complementary form of medicine really is. And finally, remember, there are many conventional medical doctors who are also homeopaths!

"Don't suppress the symptoms of your body. Disease is not an enemy to be destroyed. It is a friend to be listened to and transformed into health."

HOMEOPATHY: Q&A!

In the course of writing my articles over the years, several common themes have come up, so here are the answers to the most frequently asked questions:

Where can I buy the remedies?
You should be able to buy homeopathic remedies in your local health store. An increasing number of pharmacies now stock remedies. You can also try Nelsons Homeopathic Pharmacy in Dublin on 01 679 0451.

How much do the remedies cost?
Depending on how many you buy, the remedies should cost you between €5.00 and €10.00 – so they are very good value for money!

How long should I take the remedies?
In my experience, homeopathic healing works best if you take the remedies for two weeks, then break for two weeks, and let your body do its own healing. If you are consulting a homeopath for more chronic conditions, they will advise you on the best way to take the remedies, based on your own individual circumstances. In acute situations, for example after a shock or for an embedded thorn, you should take the remedies as often as prescribed in the relevant articles in this book.

Is homeopathic medicine safe?
Yes: homeopathic remedies are safe, non-toxic and non-addictive.

Can homeopathy be used alongside other forms of conventional medicine?
Yes.

Should I tell my doctor if I am taking homeopathic remedies?
Yes. In the same way, you should also tell your homeopath if you are taking any conventional medicines!

What form do homeopathic medicines usually take?
Homeopathic medicines are typically prescribed in small sugar pellets, but they are also available in creams and tinctures.

How are homeopathic medicines made?

Homeopathic remedies are made by a process called potentization. The relevant substance (plant, mineral, metal etc) is diluted and shaken vigorously (or successed). The process is then repeated a number of times, each time using a fraction of the resulting solution, until the desired potency is reached.

What does Potency mean?

Potency refers to how many times a remedy has been diluted. For general homeopathic usage, a 30 potency is normally used.

Where can I get more information?

Check out my website www.bredagardner.com for more information on homeopathy and its benefits. The "Useful Links" section will point you towards the Irish Society of Homeopaths, and also to some of the leading health stores and homeopathic pharmacies.

HOMEOPATHY & ENERGY IN THE BODY

Over the years, I have frequently seen the profoundly positive effect that homeopathic medicines can have on the energy levels in a person's body. This intangible force is a difficult concept to explain, which is why I love these words, written by my friend David de Roeck, on energy in the body:

"The energy of your body is in constant flux (movement). It is also changing with the mood and environment that you are in. So it is important to feed the soul with laughter as well as feed the body with food. Our bodies respond in kind to how our soul is feeling. If the soul is blocked and restrained, then our body will respond by blocking and restraining our metabolism, hence allowing the increase of toxins. As a result, we feel down and sluggish. We increase our intake of food to build ourselves up, so we believe! Yet the more we eat the worst we feel! This is cause and effect.

In this day and age, most of us will never experience true hunger, only what we let ourselves think is hunger. The blame factor comes in so strongly that we use any excuse to give in or give up to the lowest common denominator. When you believe you deserve the best, then you are on the track to receive the best, your divine light. Take responsibility for your divine path. Remember: "No response stifles effort" - so respond positively to yourself. With gifts, cards and pampering, never say you don't deserve something - always say you do. When you respond with light, laughter and love to the most important person in your life – ie YOU! – then you can respond likewise to those around you, and that will have cause and effect."

David's wonderful words coincide perfectly with my understanding of homeopathy. I believe that homeopathic medicine works on the energy of the body, right down to the DNA of the cells. Anyone who has successfully used homeopathic medicine for fatigue and stress in their life will know that the response to building up the energy levels in the body is amazing.

Some people find it difficult to understand the energy concept because it is not seen by the naked eye, or because it is not proven by science. The sun is the best way to help us understand the concept. When the sun shines, it gives us lots of energy and uplifts us. It radiates lots of energy. Another example of the energy at work – this time negative! - is a person who is an "energy drainer". We all know one! When an "energy drainer" enters the room, the atmosphere changes on another level, and we all feel and absorb their negative energy. Conversely, when they leave the room, the energy lifts, and we all breathe a collective sigh of relief - "Thank goodness they're gone!"

If you live or work with negative people or energy drainers, of if you are suffering from fatigue and stress, it important for you to protect yourself. Work on enhancing your energy, through things like positive thinking, meditation, relaxation and exercise. You can also use natural homeopathic remedies to boost your immune system, improve your energy levels, and hence bring more joy into your life. Feel it for yourself!

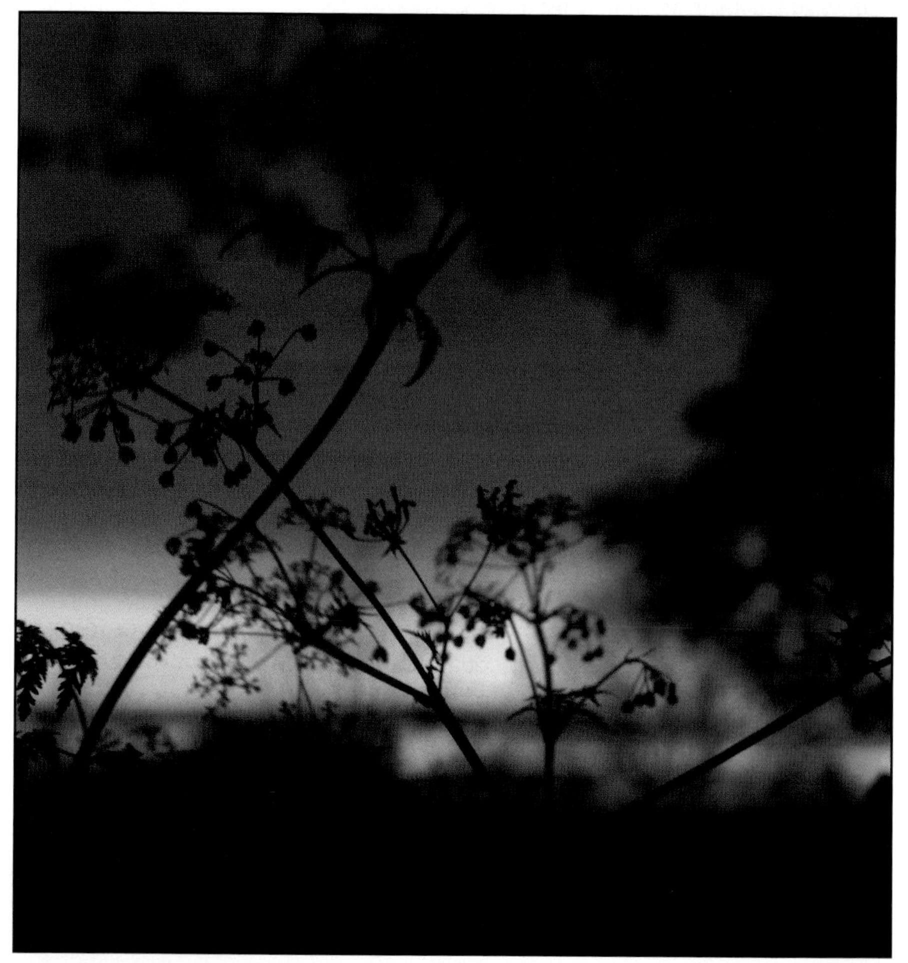

"Fears, worries and negative thoughts close the body's energies. Love opens them."

TOP TEN HOMEOPATHIC REMEDIES PART 1

As a mother and a natural health practitioner, I have been using homeopathic medicine for many years. Homeopathy is a safe, non-toxic and natural form of medicine, and it can be used in two ways: first constitutionally, to treat a person's whole body, and secondly, for first aid. I am a great believer that everybody's medical cabinet at home should contain a homeopathic first aid kit!

Remember, homeopathy is a natural healing process in which the remedies help the person to regain health by stimulating the body's own natural healing process. It does not suppress, and it enhances health – so go on, try it for yourself and see the benefits! Remember, too, that if you are in any doubt about any condition, you should seek the advice of a professional health practitioner.

As a starting point for people who would like to try out homeopathy for themselves, I have drawn up my top ten list of the most useful remedies. In time-honoured fashion, my top ten is listed in reverse order, and I will present the remaining five remedies in the next article.

10. PULSATILLA

Also known as "Wood Flower", Pulsatilla is a great remedy to use when the lymphatics (the drainage system of the body) are blocked. Pulsatilla helps to get the person's vital force moving again. Emotionally, children may be clingy, whilst adults may feel unloved, sorry for themselves and tearful. Patients are often better for fresh air and being outdoors, and worse for the warmth of a room or after over-eating fatty-type food. Pulsatilla helps people to empower themselves, to love themselves and to give love unconditionally. It also helps them to be truer to themselves.

Use for: blockages caused by ear infections, indigestion, coughs (discharges will be bland), colds and menstrual problems, depression.

9. NUX VOMICA

Nux Vomica is the number one remedy for nausea. It's a great detox remedy, especially after overindulgence, for example over-eating, over-consumption of coffee, alcohol or tobacco, or mental over-exertion. It helps people to still their minds, to live in the now, and to be more patient with both themselves and those around them.

Use for: Nausea, hangovers, IBS and conditions caused by overwork or excessive consumption of food or drink.

8. **NAT MUR**

Nat Mur is also known as Sodium Chloride, or sea salt. Patients needing this remedy often feel up one day and down the next. They feel worse for being consoled, so they keep all their worries to themselves. They may feel sad, especially in the case of women before a period. They may suffer from throbbing headaches which start in mid-morning and feel like small hammers, or from heartburn after eating, with acid rising from the stomach.

Use for: ailments that come on after emotional upsets, bereavements, losses or disappointments. Also good for respiratory infections, ie coughs and colds with post-nasal drip (colour is egg-white), sinusitis, fluid retention, headaches, chronic fatigue syndrome, insomnia, peptic ulcers and psoriasis.

7. **MERCURY**

Mercury is the number one remedy to help with abscesses, inflammation and mouth ulcers. It helps to cleanse and clear the lymphatic system: congestion and stagnation here can cause abscesses and infections. Patients may have a metallic taste in the mouth, increased flow of saliva, and a yellow-coated tongue or foul breath.

Use for: abscesses / tooth abscesses, inflammation, swollen glands, infections with green-yellow discharges, often profuse and excoriating (ie where the skin is peeling off).

6. **LYCOPODIUM**

Lycopodium is a great detox remedy, especially if the patient craves sweet things in their diet, or wakes up tired and sluggish in the morning. Other symptoms include constipation (with a feeling that the stool still remains after going to the toilet), indigestion with excessive belching, headaches (usually right sided), and a sore throat with thick yellow nasal discharge. Lycopodium raises people's self-esteem and confidence, helping them to trust more and to stop fearing the future.

Use for: digestive disorders like constipation, swollen abdomen, excessive wind and so on.

TOP TEN HOMEOPATHIC REMEDIES PART 2

Continuing my list of the most useful remedies, here are the Top 5!

5. **HYPERICUM**

Hypericum helps to relieve pain and to heal injuries to nerve-rich areas such as the toes, fingertips and gums. Falls or blows to the spine - particularly the tailbone (coccyx) – respond well to Hypericum.

Use for: Injuries (incised or lacerated wounds, scratches and abrasions). Bites, stings and puncture wounds. Bruises and burns.

4. **HEPAR SULPH**

I would call this remedy the homeopathic antibiotic. The main indicators for Hepar Sulph are infected yellow or green discharges / phlegm which freely flow from mucous membranes in the nose or ear. The patient will typically be very sensitive to cold draughts, with a peevish mood and a tendency to become angry at the slightest provocation.

Use for: Abscesses and inflammation with yellow or green discharge. Ear problems / infections, especially if throbbing or buzzing (also useful to help eliminate fluid behind the ear drums). Tooth abscess. Hoarseness and sore throats. Coughs and colds.

3. **CHAMOMILLA**

Chamomilla is a must-have remedy for mothers of teething babies. It is also an excellent remedy for children who are restless, irritable, whiney or colicky, and who want to be carried all the time. Symptoms include being worse for heat, anger and at night. Usually, only one cheek is red. Green, watery diarrhoea that looks like chopped eggs and spinach.

Use for: Teething children who are cross and complaining. Abdominal colic (gas after anger).

2. BELLADONNA

This is an excellent remedy for high temperatures characterised by sudden, violent onset and rapid progression of symptoms. Pains such as a headache can be throbbing and stabbing, and may appear and disappear suddenly, and then reappear. The patient may be worse for touch, lying down and between 3 pm and midnight. They are better for heat, sitting still and covering up. A child needing Belladonna may be delirious with fever, be restless, and may cry out during sleep because of nightmares.

Use for: Fevers, headaches, measles, coughs and colds, sore throats.

1. ARNICA

The most well-known and widely used homeopathic remedy is Arnica, so its place at number one shouldn't be too surprising! It is the first remedy to use following injury or over-exertion. The patient may be worse for touch, pressure and physical exertion, and be better for lying down.

As an example of the power of Arnica, when my son was 18 months old, he fell over and got a "duck egg" of a bruise and swelling on his forehead. I repeated a 30 potency of Arnica every 30 minutes for a few hours, and watched the miraculous reduction of the swelling before my very eyes. Arnica helps the blood to clot and to prevent internal haemorrhaging.

Use for: Bruises, sprains and strains. Abscesses and inflammation. Bleeding. Collapse and shock. Head injuries. Bites, stings and puncture wounds.

To learn more about homeopathy, you might consider coming along to my **Homeopathic First Aid & Positive Living Course** which I run twice a year in Waterford and Kilkenny. Also, I highly recommend that you purchase your own homeopathic first aid kit (available from myself or from your local health shop): the kits include a introductory booklet on the topic, and give you the opportunity to experience firsthand the wonderful benefits of this gentle, safe and effective form of healing. Finally, a reminder that if you are in any doubt about any condition, you should seek the advice of a professional health practitioner.

LIFTING DEPRESSION WITH HOMEOPATHY

Research findings published in 2006 show that homeopathy can be successfully used to help fight depression. In a national survey conducted by the Society of Homeopaths in the UK, 87% of patients who complained of mental and emotional problems reported positive change after the use of homeopathy. Some 479 patients participated in the evaluation, many of whom complained of mental and emotional symptoms as their most troublesome problem. This was the most frequent category of symptoms treated by the homeopaths participating in the trial.

"Homeopathy can prevent the downward spiral into enduring mental illness, can help patients to reduce their dependency on anti-depressants, and reduce the pressure they place on GP's," said Josephine O'Gorman, the Program Manager for CAMs (Complementary & Alternative Medicine) Integration at Waltham Forest Primary Care Trust (PCT) in the UK.

Waltham Forest PCT has successfully integrated homeopathy into its mental health strategy, using the strengths of homeopathy to treat not just mental health problems but also the physical and emotional aspects of the patient. This approach recently won them an award with the NHS.

The World Health Organisation estimates that by 2020, depression will be the second biggest health problem in the world after heart disease. Despite the amount of medicines being prescribed for depression, all of the counselling, and all of the psychotherapy, the numbers of people suffering from depression continues to rise. So what can be done?

In my early twenties, I suffered from depression myself. After taking anti-depressants for a number of years, I came to realise that they were not the answer: all they did was to suppress. I felt numb inside me. I successfully addressed and overcame my depression by using a range of complementary therapies. Today in my clinics, I also use a number of safe and effective ways alongside homeopathy and positive affirmations to help treat depression: these include advice on diet, timelines (to help discover life events that may be the root cause), and flower essences.

Homeopathy addresses the physical, mental and emotional symptoms of the patient. It also focuses on the maintaining cause of the imbalance, be it genetic, extreme sensitivity, poor diet, losses, fears or a combination of these factors: all aspects need to be addressed to help the patient to get better. Homeopaths believe that simply suppressing the symptoms is not the answer.

Many individuals testify to the benefits of homeopathy. It is estimated that 30 million people in Europe use this therapy, and the latest controlled research indicates positive outcomes from homeopathic treatment for conditions such as depression. It is my belief that we need to grow and nurture ourselves with love and natural medicines, and not suppress ourselves with fears, anxieties and toxic medicines.

HAPPY HOLIDAY REMEDIES

Q: *I'm going abroad on my holidays next month, and wondered if you could recommend any remedies to take with me. All suggestions gratefully received!*

A: Homeopathic medicines provide safe and effective treatment for a wide range of holiday ailments. Among the most common holiday complaints are gastro-intestinal problems like diarrhoea, vomiting, constipation and so on. These can be caused by new food, water or different hygiene standards, especially in places like India, Africa or South America. As ever, prevention is better than cure. It's best to avoid tap water and drink only bottled water. Also remember to avoid foods that may be troublesome, like ice-creams, ice cubes, milks, salads washed in untreated water and so on. Finally, if you are in any doubt about any ailment, you should consult a health professional. But you specifically asked about useful holiday homeopathic remedies, so here are my recommendations:

ACONITE: for fright, shock, anxiety and panic attacks: great to use if you suffer these symptoms when flying.

APIS: for insect bites, stings and stinging pains, swellings and acute cystitis.

ARNICA: for injuries, bruising, trauma, also excellent for jet lag.

ARSENICUM: for vomiting and / or diarrhoea, burns or burning pains, also anxiety with illness.

BELLADONNA: for fevers and inflammations, pains that are hot / throbbing in nature, also overheating, ie sunburn.

BRYONIA: gastric flu (vomiting / diarrhoea) with marked irritability.

CANTHARSIS: burns or burning-type pains with restlessness, also an acute remedy for cystitis.

CITRONELLA ESSENTIAL OIL: not a remedy, but added to sun cream can help to repel mosquitoes.

CARBO VEG: for altitude sickness when mountaineering, also great for sleep apnoea and snoring, as it helps to oxygenate the body.

COCCULUS: for car and sea-sickness with nausea, dizziness and / or diarrhoea.

HEPAR SULPH: also known as the homeopathic antibiotic, excellent for tooth abscesses with swollen red gums that may ooze pus. Also great for ear, nose and throat infections.

HYPERICUM: for accidents and injuries to the nerves and nerve-rich areas (eg fingers, toes, eyes, lips), insect bites with sharp shooting pains. Can also be applied in cream form to treat open cuts and wounds.

NAT MUR: for cold sores that come up due to exposure to the sun. Also good for heartburn.

NUX VOMICA: for stomach pain and nausea (including motion sickness) that are better for vomiting. Also good for when you have eaten or drunk too much.

PULSATILLA: for nausea and vomiting associated with over-indulgence of fatty type foods and ice-cream.

RHUS TOX: for cold sores that are worse for damp, wet weather, with cracks in the lips. Also great for easing the itch of and aiding recovery from chicken pox.

These remedies are available in 6C or 30 potency from health shops (I would recommend the latter potency), and can be taken approximately every 2 – 4 hours depending on the intensity of the symptoms. If you don't get an improvement after three doses, consider another remedy. There is no problem repeating the remedy frequently if needed. However, if you notice an improvement soon after taking a remedy, then it's best to stop taking it. Homeopathy works by stimulating the body's own natural healing mechanisms, and if there's an improvement, then that process has started to work!

I sell homeopathic first aid remedy kits in my clinics: see the useful addresses section at the back of this book for details of other outlets.

7
WHICH HOMEOPATHIC PERSONALITY ARE YOU?

INTRODUCTION TO HOMEOPATHIC PERSONALITIES

Q: *My husband recently attended your clinic and said he was amazed at how accurately you described his personality, despite not knowing him. You told him he had an "Aurum" personality, always going for gold, and that he was too much of a perfectionist. This describes him perfectly! I'm fascinated and would love to know more: also, are there other different personalities? By the way, he is doing really well since he came to see you!*

A: Thank you for your kind and interesting letter! For every consultation, I use a combination of iridology (study of the iris) and muscle testing to help me identify any imbalances in the body, and often I find there is a homeopathic remedy that describes the different layers of the client's personality – "Aurum" in your husband's case. In order to help heal themselves, clients often have to remove one or more layers, and homeopathic remedies can help in this process: again in your husband's case, Aurum will help him to accept himself better, to be more comfortable with himself, to stop comparing himself to others, and to realise that perfection isn't always needed!

There are eight remedies that I use most commonly in my clinics, and each one has a "state" or "layer" associated with it. The layers or states include fear, anxiety, shock, bereavement and so on: and each can be responsible for imbalances in the body like migraines, fatigue, irritable bowel, depression and so on – you name it! As an example, a client presents with panic attacks which, on further investigation, began after a near death experience. This was a real shock to the system, and to treat the panic attacks, the cause – or layer – needs to be removed to help the body heal. In this example, Aconite would be the prescribed remedy. We all have many layers, meaning we may slip in and out of the different homeopathic personalities.

So here's the list of my eight most commonly prescribed remedies, and the conditions they help to treat:

- **ACONITE: to alleviate shock and fears in the body.**
- **ARSENICUM: to stop anxiety and worry, and to regain peace in the cells of the body.**
- **AURUM: to bring more joy into your life, and to help you understand**

that you do not need to aim for perfection every time.

- **LYCOPODIUM: to overcome a lack of confidence and self-esteem, and to help you to trust more in the flow of life.**
- **NAT MUR: to release sorrow and sadness from the cells due to loss or disappointment.**
- **NUX VOMICA: to be more patient and to live in the now.**
- **PULSATILLA: to regain and feel more comfortable with your own power.**
- **SEPIA: to help you find your purpose in life and to tune into your creativity.**

In the following articles, I describe each of these remedies in more depth, covering the mental, physical and emotional aspects of the homeopathic "personality" associated with each remedy. I also cover the reasons why people move into these states, and the positive results the remedies can bring. If you think the descriptions apply to you, ask in your local health store or pharmacy for a 30 potency of the relevant remedy. Take twice daily for two weeks and then let your body do the healing. Please remember not to take the remedies for more than two weeks at a time - after 14 days, the body needs to be able to take over the healing process on its own. Otherwise, you may find yourself taking on more symptoms of the remedy instead of healing the matching symptoms! Finally, remember that all homeopathic medicine can be taken alongside conventional treatments: your informed GP will reassure you!

THE ACONITE PERSONALITY: RELEASE THE FEAR

Aconite is an extremely effective remedy to release shocks and fears in the body.

Who needs Aconite?

A person who needs Aconite may suffer from fear or anxiety of mind and body. This fear may have commenced following a severe shock or fright to the system. Examples of such shocks and frights include hearing bad news, a death in the family, a near death experience, or invasive surgery (many people are terrified of surgery and worry they won't survive the ordeal – ditto with fear of flying). All of these shocks and frights can lead to an Aconite state.

Physical Ailments: Heart palpitations, vertigo / dizzy spells, fainting, headache, urgent desire to urinate more, feeling of choking on swallowing (feels as if something is stuck in the throat). Hoarse, dry, croupy cough, insomnia and nervousness. Rheumatic complaints. Tonsillitis. Heart attacks. Chest infections. Angina.

Mental & Emotional Ailments: Panic attacks, fears crowds or even crossing the street, may become housebound. Pains are intolerable, person worries a lot. Restlessness, tossing and turning. Person may be nervous and is startled easily. Feels as if thoughts are coming from the stomach. Afraid of the dark. May suffer from migraines or anxious dreams. Phobias, especially fear of death.

Positive results from Aconite

Aconite is the number one remedy to help alleviate panic attacks, and is also the main remedy for treating the early stages of croup. By helping to remove fear and shock from the system, Aconite heals the conditions associated with those fears and shocks. It can also release a deep-seated fright or shock that has been held in the body for a lifetime: in some instances, the person may have forgotten or blocked out the cause of the shock, and may not even be aware that they are still holding on to it.

In my experience, fear is often stored in the kidneys (this accounts for the desire to urinate frequently), and Aconite provides excellent support to both the kidneys and bladder, thus alleviating physical conditions in these areas. Aconite also helps people to be more relaxed, both about themselves and about their lives. It helps people lose their fear of death, and to enjoy life more.

THE ARSENICUM PERSONALITY: STOP WORRYING!

Arsenicum is an excellent remedy to stop anxiety and worry, and to help you regain peace in the cells of your body.

Perhaps you are a worrier. Or maybe you know someone who worries constantly. Worriers worry about everything: money, poverty, deadlines, exams and exam results, their own or a loved one's health, flying, death, leaving the backdoor unlocked, world peace, nuclear war: the list is endless! An anxious Arsenicum personality has the capacity to become afraid of – or to worry about – just about anything! They often worry about things that in all likelihood will never happen. And they even worry when they have nothing to worry about!

Who needs Arsenicum?

People who need Arsenicum are often insecure and may suffer from a lot of anxiety. In the early stages of this "homeopathic state", the most marked emotional symptoms are irritability, criticism and discontent. As the insecurity increases, the person may develop frightening panic or anxiety attacks, with great restlessness (they can't keep still for a moment), together with a strong desire for company and reassurance. All of this may have arisen from a minor worrying thought which suddenly becomes overwhelming, taking over the person's whole being and resulting in conditions like insomnia or tightness in the chest.

People needing this remedy are often extremely fastidious, obsessively putting everything in order. This may be due to an overpowering need to be in control at all times, to help them to feel more secure. The stress that accumulates over time may cause the person to "break" quite suddenly, resulting in a nervous breakdown. Their anxiety often becomes overwhelming, meaning they cease to function rationally.

Physical Ailments: Stomach / chest complaints: angina, gastritis, peptic ulcers, colitis (with extreme burning). Asthma, worse between midnight and 2 am. Food poisoning. Thirsty for small, frequent sips of water. Insomnia, especially difficulty in dropping off to sleep. Eczema with dry skin and intense burning and itching.

Mental & Emotional Ailments: Tremendous anxiety often with great restlessness. Panic attacks, especially after midnight. Constantly needs reassurance from their doctor. Compulsive disorders, eg constant house cleaning or washing of hands. Depression to the point of contemplating suicide. Anorexia nervosa.

Positive results from Arsenicum

Arsenicum is the number one remedy to help relieve anxiety, depression and insomnia. It helps to stop worriers from worrying so much! It also aids in the cleansing of all the mucous membranes in the body, and hence facilitates the healing of ulcers, colitis, asthma and skin ailments. I often prescribe this remedy in my clinics to help clients to heal themselves on their own, and to move on with their lives, rather than staying stuck in a rut.

THE AURUM PERSONALITY: GOING FOR GOLD!

Do you take life too seriously? Are you always striving for perfection, always going for gold? Do you have an over-developed sense of duty, meaning you feel guilty if things are not going to plan or going your way? If so, read on – you may have an Aurum personality.

Who needs Aurum?

The Aurum child grows up sensing that love is only forthcoming from his parents when he does his best to please them. This in turn can lead to a seriousness and a lack of spontaneity in the child, which often progresses to feelings of depression and despair even before the child becomes an adult.

Aurum is a remedy that often suits people who are very intense, ambitious, idealistic, who want to be the best and who set very high goals for themselves. If these (sometimes unrealistic) goals are not achieved, the Aurum personality can go through a period of tremendous irritability and violent or even suicidal ideas and thoughts.

Physical Ailments: A wide range which arise after business reversals or humiliation: may include headaches, back problems, bone pains and so on. Angina or chest pains, worse in the evening or on ascending stairs – sensation as if the heart or chest is encased in armour. Palpitations, worse at night, worse from emotions and anxiety. Chronic fatigue syndrome. Heart disease.

Mental & Emotional Ailments: Outbursts of anger and extreme irritability. Fears failure and heights. May wake up 3 – 4 hours after falling asleep. Severe, chronic insomnia. May feel low and depressed.

Positive results from Aurum

I have used Aurum to help people to bring more joy and love into their heart, blood circulation and hence into their lives. Above all, Aurum is an uplifting remedy. It seems to relieve the heavy burden of responsibility and pressure that they put on themselves. Suddenly they see life differently. They become more gracious and more accepting of what they have, rather than focusing on what they "should have" or "must do." Remember that when you positively accept the "I am's" and the "I have's" in your life rather than the guilt-inducing "I should's" or "I must's", then you will experience greater joy from living in the now.

A good friend of mine who works in the medical profession reckoned that most of the profoundly depressed patients in the psychiatric wards would benefit from this homeopathic remedy, to help them with their symptoms of emotional flatness, despair of ever recovering, sense of wretchedness (and hence deserving punishment), slowness of thought and feeling that nothing can get through to them. On a brighter note, Aurum can help people to be grateful for the positive aspects of their lives.

THE LYCOPODIUM PERSONALITY: TRUST MORE

Lycopodium is a great remedy to overcome a lack of confidence and self-esteem, and to help you to trust more in the flow of life.

Who needs Lycopodium?

A person in a Lycopodium state feels a lack of self-worth, and may become very shy, introverted, soft, and a loner. They can be very anxious about their health, and have fears about being alone at night, or about death or survival. Often, however, their main fear is people in authority. On the flip side, however, they themselves can be very domineering, and behave very arrogantly towards family and those with less authority. They like to be in control at all times.

Their fears stem from a lack of trust in the flow of life, and indeed a fear of what the future may hold – they often ask themselves the hypothetical question "What if?" Their pessimistic thoughts take over, bombard their heads and make their outlook very negative.

Physical Ailments: Fatigue worse on waking up and between 4 - 8 pm. Craves sweets / sweet things. Loud rumbling in the abdomen. Bloated and distended abdomen. Heartburn with sour burping. Asthma with chronic dry, tickling cough. Pneumonia, especially right sided. Psoriasis.

Mental & Emotional Ailments: Issues of self-esteem and low confidence. Bullying, domineering, arrogant behaviour towards family or people with less authority. Fears: losing control, the future, people, public speaking, being alone at night. Anxiety around health. Dyslexia: reverses letters and words when reading or speaking. Averse to company yet dreads being alone.

Positive results from Lycopodium

I frequently use Lycopodium in my clinics. It can help to overcome a sluggish liver: indeed it's a great remedy for the liver and gastro-intestinal organs. Everything we eat and drink goes through the liver. If the energy of the liver is not good, then motivation is not there, and hence people can become sluggish in both mind and body. Because it helps the liver to function more efficiently, Lycopodium boosts people's energy, reduces fatigue and helps them to be more positive in their thoughts. Remember, what you fear most, you often attract, so it is important to trust in the flow of life and stop the need to be in control of everything. With Lycopodium, you might just find synchronicity and greater happiness come into your life, enabling you to find joy in the simple, small pleasures that are already present in your life.

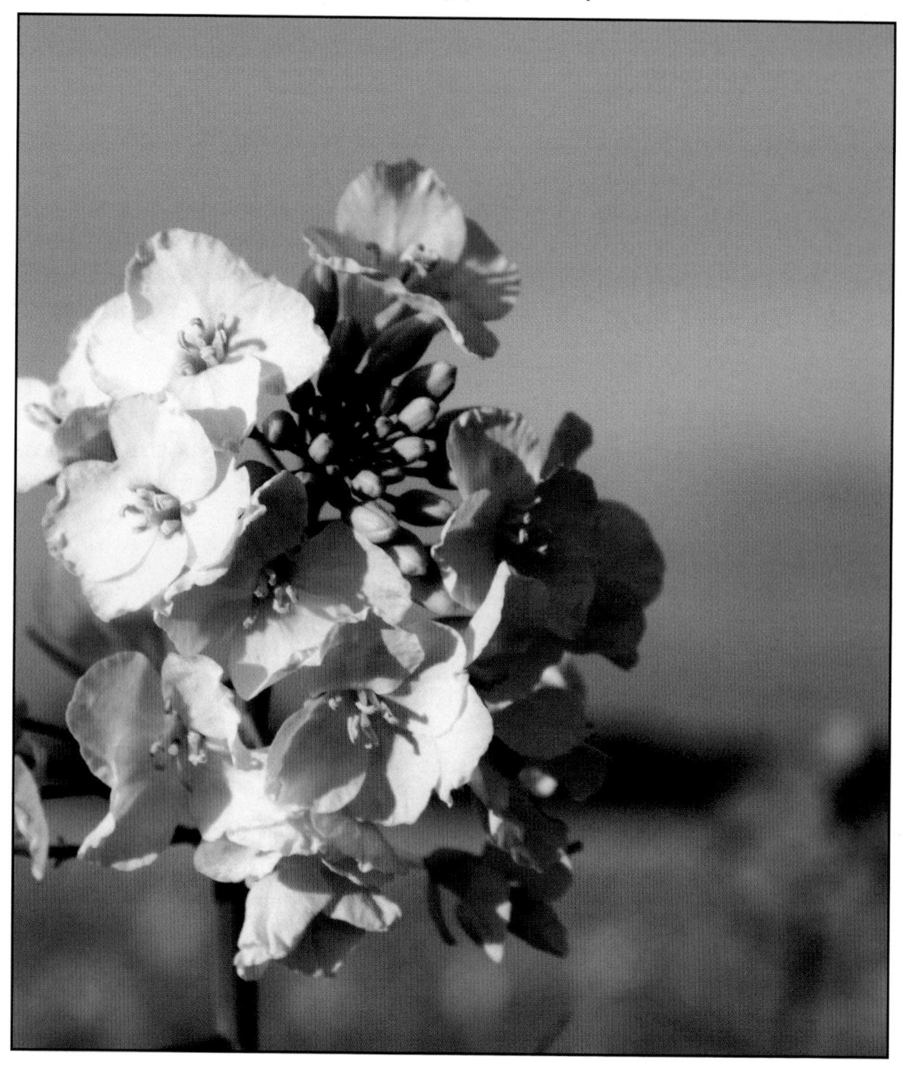

"To trust the universe it is necessary to be vulnerable."

THE NAT MUR PERSONALITY: END THE SORROW & SADNESS

Nat Mur helps to release sorrow and sadness from the cells due to loss or disappointment.

Who needs Nat Mur?

Everyone has either experienced - or knows someone who has experienced – a deep hurt, disappointment or sadness in their life, caused by a loss. This sense of loss can come from many quarters. It may be the loss of a loved one, of a job, of a relationship, a friend or a pet. Or it may be a loss of identity, of good health, of independence, from a child leaving home, of innocence / child-hood, of reputation ... the list really is endless. Nat Mur - with its associated sense of loss - is by far the most common homeopathic state / personality that I come across in my clinics.

Physical Ailments: Headaches worse at 10 am or from 10 am to 3 pm. Headaches or dizzy spells (vertigo) in schoolchildren. Bitten fingernails. Sinusitis, discharge from nose is egg white. Lower back pain. Colds begin-ning with sneezing. Cold sores. Twitches or tremors, especially on face and head. Thyroid conditions. Sensation of a lump in the throat. May crave salt. Palpitations at night, worse for lying on left side. Chronic fatigue syndrome. Depression (sighs a lot). Insomnia. Multiple sclerosis. Nephritis (inflammation of one or both kidneys). Peptic ulcers. Psoriasis.

Mental & Emotional Ailments: Due to the grief held in the cells, may be very sensitive to criticism or insults: can be angry, overreact to situations, take things too personally, and find it hard to forgive. May put a wall around themselves to avoid further hurt, and thus may appear closed or even hard. Can become very serious, overly responsible and perfectionist. Always on time, compulsive and likes to control their environment. Dwells a lot on past unpleasant memories. Likes to cry alone. Fears robbers or people breaking into their house. Fears storms or heights.

Positive results from Nat Mur

Nat Mur helps people to heal the losses, hurts and disappointments in their lives, giving them the opportunity to move on. Nat Mur personalities are often up one day and down the next: their symptoms can change on alternate days. By helping to remove blockages in the body's cells, Nat Mur helps to get people's energy flowing again, and thus it can shift many of the ailments described above. It makes people believe in the flow of life again, and allows them to love unconditionally, by breaking down the protective wall around them. It helps people to talk and communicate their true feelings. In many cases, people do not want to go there, because of the pain – but Nat Mur is very good at releasing the blocked tears. Remember, for every tear shed, a day is added to your life.

THE NUX VOMICA PERSONALITY: LIVE IN THE NOW

Nux Vomica helps you to be more patient and to live in the now.

Who needs Nux Vomica?

Do you know anybody who is impatient, competitive and ambitious? The major focus in their life is to work and to achieve. Such people can be very confident - arrogant even - and often they are compulsive not just in their work, but also in all aspects of their life. The pathology of the Nux Vomica personality focuses on the gastro intestinal tract. Indeed, this personality often craves stimulant type food and drink such as spicy or fatty foods, alcohol, coffee and cigarettes.

Physical Ailments: IBS. Constipation with constant, ineffectual urging for stool - or the opposite, ie urgency for diarrhoea. Haemorrhoids. Gastritis with pains from alcohol abuse or from over-eating. Acute colic: kidney or gall stones with cramping pains, better for heat and worse for touch. Insomnia: wakes up especially between 2 and 3 am due to thoughts about work, exams or tasks to achieve.

Mental & Emotional Ailments: Irritable, ambitious and driven. Easily offended and can lose temper easily. Anger at contradiction from others. Tendency to break things from anger and frustration. Impatient: hates waiting in lines or in traffic (can suffer from road rage). Competitive. Workaholic. Fastidious, can become especially angry if objects are not in their proper place. Their minds think very fast and can leap from one idea to the next. Slow workers can irritate them.

The Nux Vomica child is irritable and often suffers from colic or colitis. At school age the child is extremely competitive about sports and exam results, and they can be terrible losers. The child may be rude towards siblings, parents and peers, and may lack concentration and focus due to day-dreaming.

Positive results from Nux Vomica

Nux Vomica is the number one remedy for irritable bowel syndrome (IBS), and helps to treat the associated spasms, cramps, burping and belching which are so prevalent with this condition. It helps people to be more patient with themselves and to be more tolerant of others. By calming the nerves, it helps people to concentrate better and to be more focussed. And by calming the nerves, it can also aid the relaxation of the colon and over-ride IBS-type symptoms. Nux Vomica helps people to get the right balance in their lives between work, family and self-contentment.

Nux Vomica is a wonderful remedy for getting people to live in the now. With this remedy, when they apply themselves to a job, they actually see it through without distraction, and without becoming frustrated at the perceived failings of both themselves and those around them. Otherwise, they may find that they are present in body but not in their thoughts which may be elsewhere – in other words daydreaming.

Finally, Nux Vomica is a wonderful detox remedy for the mind and body: many of you may know it as the number one hangover remedy!

THE PULSATILLA PERSONALITY: EMPOWER YOURSELF

Pulsatilla helps you to regain and feel more comfortable with your own power. Pulsatilla cleans the lymphatic system (the drainage system of the body) and cleanses the blood.

Who needs Pulsatilla?

Are you someone who finds it difficult to say no? Who is always giving of yourself, but who finds it very hard to receive – even a simple compliment? Do you sometimes feel yourself to be a victim, and hence blame everyone around you - or your current circumstances - for your problems? If this sounds like you, then you are a Pulsatilla personality!

Physical Ailments: blocked lymphatic system resulting in conditions such as tonsillitis, ear infections with a creamy white or yellowy green discharge, and PMT (especially breast tenderness and tearfulness before and after periods). May crave stodgy-type comfort foods like chocolate, cheese, cake, biscuits, ice-cream etc. Worse for fatty-type foods yet may crave them (eg pork, ice-cream, milk and cheese). Bowels may be very loose, rumbling and watery. No two stools alike. May also have mucous discharge. Constipation or conversely diarrhoea. Dry cough in the evening and at night – needs to sit upright to get relief. Loose cough in the morning with lots of phlegm. Bad smell from the breath.

Mental & Emotional Ailments: Mood is changeable - they are, loving one moment and very demanding the next. They weep easily and fear abandonment, rejection and not being accepted. They are always giving of themselves even when they don't want to, because they want to be accepted. This can lead to a feeling of resentment, which comes out as blame. People in this state are always rescuing others because they see the victim in them – when what they really need to do is rescue themselves. May crave sugar, cigarettes, alcohol, cheese and processed foods, all of which can block their lymphatic system. As a child, may suffer from tantrums, be very clingy and want to be held.

Positive results from Pulsatilla

Pulsatilla helps people to be comfortable with their own power. It helps them to love and respect themselves more, and by doing this, they will gain more love and respect from the people around them. It makes people more positive and optimistic, by lifting their mood. It helps them to overcome social shyness and make friends more easily. It enhances the immune system and reduces the cravings for low energy foods.

THE SEPIA PERSONALITY: FIND YOUR PURPOSE IN LIFE

Sepia helps you to find your purpose in life and to tune into your creativity.

Who needs Sepia?

Do you always seem to be bored, fatigued, indifferent to your loved ones, and easily offended? If so, you may need Sepia. Sepia is sometimes known as "the housewife's remedy", for whom the monotony of always "doing" never seems to stop – endless cooking, washing, tidying up, ironing, child-rearing and so on! But in many ways, Sepia is a man's remedy too – for example a builder or businessman who is always working too hard and never has any time to enjoy himself.

Physical Ailments: Chronic fatigue syndrome. Raynaud's syndrome (hands and feet very cold). Cystitis / stress incontinence on coughing. Endometriosis / hot flushes / menopause. Migraines. Miscarriages. Pre-menstrual syndrome. Psoriasis / dry skin / vitiligo / ringworm. May feel cold even when in a warm room.

Mental & Emotional Ailments: Marked irritability, depression and indifference – any demand made by the family is viewed as a further burden and met with anger. May find themselves shrieking at the children and cannot control their temper. Often feels guilty about and afraid of their internal changes, and can present themselves with tearfulness and desperation. Ultimately can lose their connection to others and no longer feel remorse for their behaviour. Because of their detachment, they can see clearly into the weaknesses of those around them, and will lash out with cutting, accurate, sarcastic and hurtful words. May crave chocolate.

Positive results from Sepia

Sepia helps people to find their own inner sanctuary space. By this I mean that it helps you to tune into and find time for whatever you really love to do for yourself, for example painting, music, exercise, dancing, or just allowing yourself time to relax and read your favourite book. Sepia is also a great hormone balancing remedy, especially if a low sex drive is present with a laxness in the body's tissues, ie constipation, prolapses, varicose veins and so on.

Sepia can help to lift people out of their despair and depression. It helps to motivate them to try and find time for themselves. I have even seen Sepia help to save marriages. In cases where the wife or husband has become indifferent or has fallen out of love, Sepia can reduce the irritability and despair, and hence allow them to connect more to just "being" rather than constantly "doing." It helps them to relax more and achieve what they wish to do, with least effort and with more fun and joy in their lives. Finally, if you are a chocoholic, Sepia can help to reduce your craving for chocolate!

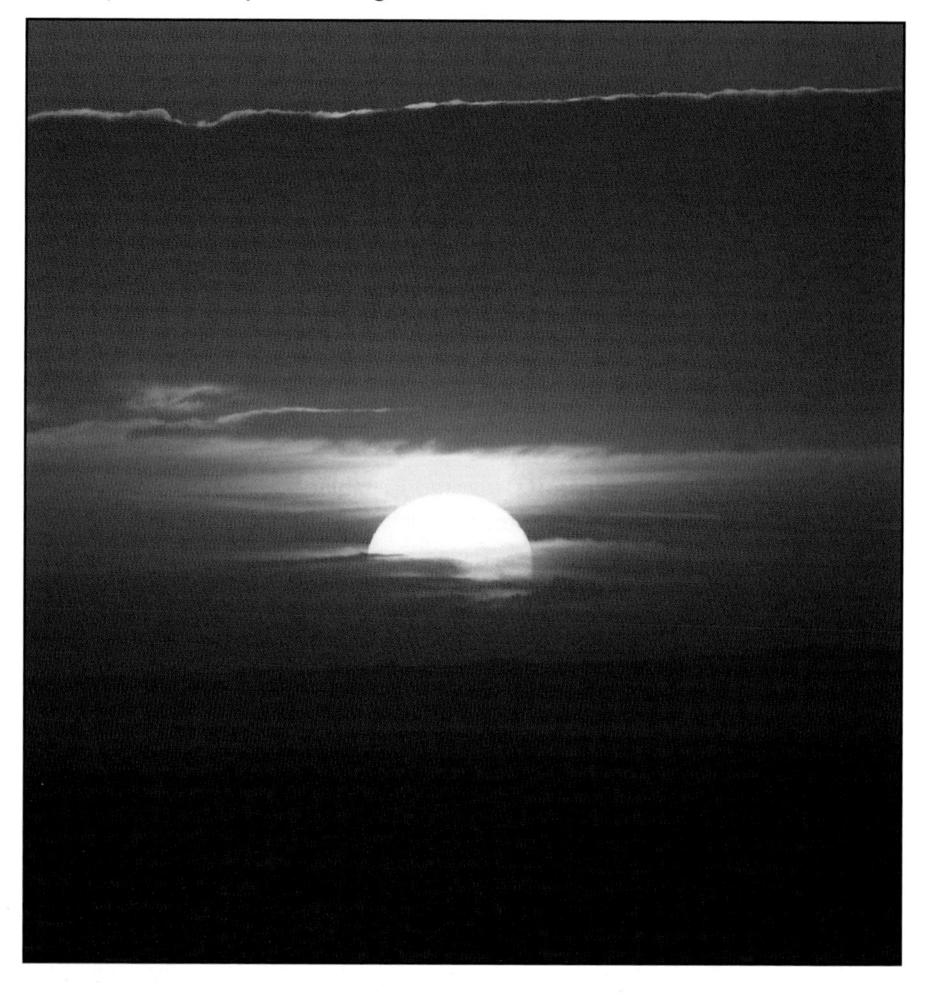

"Imagination is creation. It is where anything is possible."

8
POSITIVE LIVING

DON'T WORRY – BE HAPPY!

In my clinics, I hear the following questions on a daily basis: "How can I stop worrying? Why can't I let go of the past instead of carrying a burden around with me?" As the song goes, the answer is "Don't Worry – Be Happy!"

Guilt and worry are perhaps the most common forms of distress in our culture today. With guilt, you focus on a past event, feel dejected or angry about something that you did or said, and use up your present moments being occupied with feelings over the past behaviour. And with worry, you use up those valuable "nows", becoming obsessed about a future event that may even not happen. Whether you are looking backwards or forwards, the result is always the same: you are throwing away the present moment.

Author Robert Burdette's "Golden Day" is really "today": the central theme is to live in the now. He sums up the folly of guilt and worry with these words:

"There are two days in the week about which and upon which I never worry. Two carefree days, kept sacredly free from fear and apprehension. One of these days is yesterday … and the other day I do not worry about is tomorrow."

Guilt is the most useless aspect of our emotional behaviour. Why? Because by definition you are immobilised in the present over something that has already taken place, and no amount of guilt can ever change history. Instead of continually going back, keep working on your joy and happiness in the present moment, and accept yourself as you are. Nobody is perfect, so stop comparing yourself to anyone else.

Just as our society fosters guilt, so it encourages worry. We equate worrying with caring. If you care about someone, so the message goes, then you are bound to worry about them. Worry is endemic in our culture. But not one moment of worry will make things any better. In fact, worrying will very likely make you less effective in dealing with the present, as worry creates unnecessary stress and anxiety in our lives.

In my clinic in Kilkenny, the following Irish prayer hangs on the wall. Use it to help you overcome worry in your life.

AN IRISH PRAYER

Take time to work: it is the price of success
Take time to meditate: it is the source of power
Take time to play: it is the secret to perpetual youth
Take time to read: it is the way to knowledge
Take time to be friendly: it is the road to happiness
Take time to laugh: it is the music of the soul
Take time to love and be loved, at all times in your life.

GUILT & WORRY: LET GO!

In my article entitled "Don't Worry – Be Happy", I wrote about guilt and worry, and in this article I outline more strategies on how to overcome these most negative of emotions.

In many respects, guilt and worry are the opposite of love. They are both negative energies that can and do affect the weak areas in our bodies. In some people this can mean the spine, leading to aches and pains in the back area. With others, guilt and worry can affect the heart, because joy is stagnant in the blood and not moving efficiently, potentially bringing with it problems in circulation, such as high cholesterol, high blood pressure or even in some cases heart attacks. Remember the heart doesn't "attack" us – we can allow it to happen through our emotions, be it guilt or excessive worrying.

A book I would highly recommend on this topic is "Your Erroneous Zones" by Dr Wayne Dyer. He makes the following points:

Begin to view the past as something that can never be changed, no matter how you feel about it. Accept that any guilt you choose to feel will not make the past any different.

Accept yourself and stop the self-criticism. The more you accept yourself and stop putting yourself down, the better other people will accept you too. You will not then need other people's approval either.

Keep a guilt journal, and make a note of what you are avoiding in the present with this agonising over the past. Make a list of all the bad things you have ever done. Give yourself guilt points for each on a scale of one to ten. Add up your score and see if it makes any difference whether your tally is a hundred, a thousand or a million points in the present. The present moment is still the same and all your guilt is a complete waste of time. Burn the sheet afterwards to symbolically get rid of the guilt in your life.

Say the following positive affirmation daily morning and evening to help retain more positive thoughts in your head and to help alleviate any stress and dis-ease entering your body:

"I ask that all the effects of my mistakes be undone in all directions of time, and I now release all guilt completely. I love my true self from head to toe."

So release the negativity of guilt and worry, and allow joy and happiness to flow through your body once again. Remember, you are worth it!

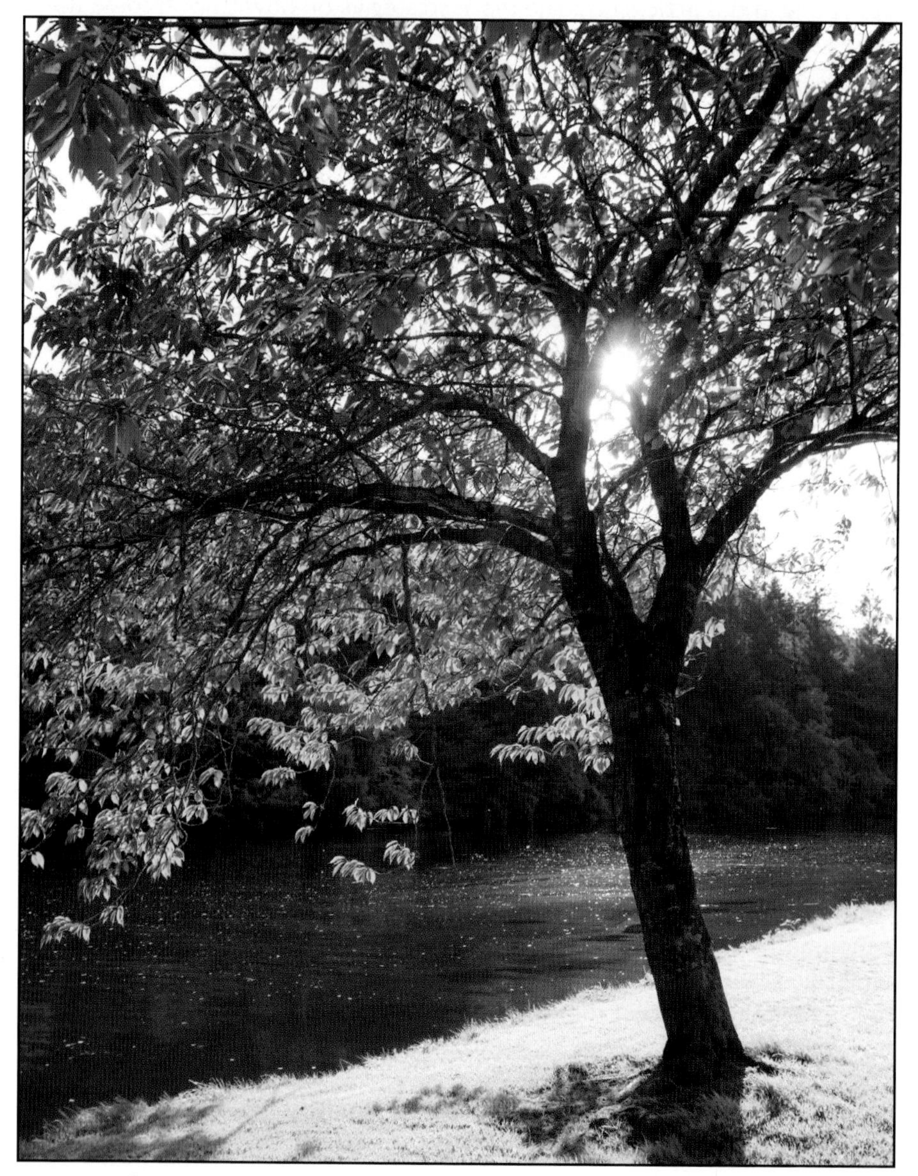

"When you let go and trust, something better comes to take its place."

INNER SANCTUARY – PART 1

In these heady days of the Celtic Tiger, most people lead extremely hectic lives. We each have a raft of responsibilities: not just our families and our work, but also our friendships and our social, community and political responsibilities. Even our recreational activities often take up much of our attention and energy. We are very involved in what is outside of us.

Most of us need to balance this focus on "the outside" by taking some time to go within ourselves. Each of us needs to get back in contact with our spirit, with our inner, creative source.

I believe that each of us has a deep sense of truth within us - the guiding force that can lead us through our lives. But when we spend most of our time looking outside ourselves – for example worrying about what other people think about us, or thinking "I must stay in this job even though I hate it, because I need the money" – then we are in danger of losing contact with the creative source within us.

It is a sad fact that most of us have not been educated to believe in that inner, intuitive knowingness. Rather, we have been brought up to follow "outside" laws: other people's rules, other people's concepts of what is right and wrong for us, other people's ideas of what we need to be doing. As a result, we lose touch with the very core of our being. If you spend too much time looking outwards, then there will always be a part of you that will want to go "within" to find the answers.

Instead of rushing around all the time, we need to take time to cultivate contact with our inner, wise self. Step off the merry-go-round for once, and appreciate the value of peace, calm and silence! We need to re-educate ourselves to pay attention to that part of us that really knows. It helps if we can begin to put aside some regular time for this – even if it is just a few minutes each day, or even a few minutes each week. We need this time to switch off our minds, learn to relax our bodies and move into the deeper awareness that exists within each of us. But doing so takes practice, patience and support. The form your inner sanctuary takes is up to you: meditation, deep breathing, or taking a walk in nature are all examples of how we can get in touch with our inner self.

For many people, the route to their inner sanctuary is by practising deep breathing exercises every morning, breathing in positive energy, and breathing out fears, worries and negative energy. After a while, this becomes a natural part of your life. Combine this simple technique with walks in nature and it will become even more recharging.

Another way of stepping off the merry-go-round is to read a new poem out loud every day, to yourself, or your partner or family. So why not pop along to your local library and choose a book with your favourite poems?

INNER SANCTUARY – PART 2

Q: *I am a stressed-out housewife with three young children aged 4, 6 and 10 years old. A couple of weeks ago, you wrote about finding your inner sanctuary – some hope for me! I seem to be always on the go, with school runs, club runs, meals, homework – the list is endless! I never get a break, and don't seem to be able to find time to be still. Please help! – is there anything you can suggest to assist me in finding my inner sanctuary?*

A: From personal experience, I know exactly what you are going through! I know that it's not easy, but you can and must make yourself a sanctuary area, with a comfortable chair that supports your back. Set your alarm five minutes earlier in the morning, and try the following:

- **Light a candle and put on some relaxing, soothing music**
- **Sit and be still for five minutes**
- **Breathe in through your nose to the count of 4, then pause for 2 seconds, before slowly breathing out through your mouth. As you inhale, imagine you are breathing in positive energy and happiness for the day. As you exhale, imagine you are breathing out all your worries, fears and unwanted thoughts.**

Don't worry about your kids: they will soon learn that this is Mum's quiet time and space, and will respect it. Kids adjust easily. These 5 minutes will help to ground you more, stop your head spinning, and will help you to achieve twice as much in the day with less effort.

It's important that you get a break from the children at least one evening during the week and possibly for a few hours at the weekend. Get your husband, partner, family or friends to help, or if necessary, do swaps with other parents. With this precious time, create space for yourself on something you love to do, for example dance classes, photography, walks in nature etc. Don't feel one bit guilty: you need your own space, so create it and enjoy it. You will find that with the help of the 5 minute deep breathing technique in the morning, plus exercise, plus doing something you really love, your mood will lift, and more joy and happiness will come into your life. Enjoy!

OVERCOMING FATIGUE

Q: *I find myself suffering increasingly from fatigue, especially in the mornings. I just feel so lethargic – it takes me at least half an hour to get going. I am in my 30's and have a stressful job in sales. My diet could be better – I crave sweet things like chocolate and cake. Can you give me some suggestions on how to get more energy?*

A:The energy in our bodies is in constant movement. It also changes with our mood and the environment in which we find ourselves. In your case, there is clearly a block in the flow of energy in your body. Your blockage – or fatigue – could be the result of many factors: diet, lifestyle (working or partying too hard!), lack of sleep, an undiagnosed illness or allergy, your environment, negative thinking, dehydration, relationship issues, unhappiness and depression, a lack of fun, laughter and joy, too little exercise, no sense of direction in your life – the list goes on!

My first piece of advice would be to take some time to reflect on your life. Sometimes we can't see the wood for the trees, and there might be an obvious cause for your fatigue once you take the time to stop and think about it. Are you getting enough sleep? (at least eight hours). Is your work / life balance all wrong? Are you drinking enough water? (at least eight glasses a day). Your diet might also be responsible. Eating chocolate and cakes is like putting petrol on a fire - the flames burn brightly but are soon extinguished. You need to include slow-burning, long-lasting foods in your diet, rather than eating things which only give you a temporary boost.

In my clinics, I see many people with fatigue, and one thing they often have in common is over sensitivity. They take everything too personally, and make assumptions that simply aren't true. They are also sensitive to electromagnetic stress from man-made electrics like mobiles, computers, pylons, fluorescent lights and so on, and suffer from static shocks (eg when touching a car door). This can all mean they are living too much in their heads - with too many thoughts with no space in between! - and simply need to be more grounded. Walking in nature, doing more exercise and meditation are all simple and effective ways to ground yourself. You can also use crystals to protect yourself from electromagnetic stress.

I wonder if you are unhappy in your job. Our bodies respond in kind to how our soul is feeling. If the soul is blocked and restrained, then our bodies respond by blocking and restraining our metabolism, hence increasing the level of toxins in our circulatory systems. As a result we feel down and sluggish. So if you are unhappy in your job, perhaps it is time to move on.

Remember: "When you believe you deserve the best, then you are on track to receive the best." Take more responsibility for your health and well-being, and enjoy life to its fullest potential.

You could also try the homeopathic remedies Lycopodium and Pulsatilla. Lycopodium helps to detox the liver, and can also improve your energy levels in the morning and make you more motivated. Pulsatilla helps to clean out the lymphatic system, and can empower you to take more responsibility to make changes in your life to make you happier and healthier (eg by changing your diet or job). At the moment you see yourself as the victim, so get out of that mindset and become more empowered to do something positive about your situation!

OVERCOMING LONELINESS

Loneliness is a major problem in Western society, as a result of the difficulties we have in getting close to others and sustaining intimate relationships. Instead, our lifestyles offer endless activities in pursuit of pleasure, from clubbing to the movies – but they only distract momentarily from a sense of isolation. Alienation stems from a lack of connection with others, and leaves you feeling separate, even in company. You can suffer from inner loneliness whether your life is full and busy or seemingly empty.

You feel alone when you close your heart to yourself. This can happen when you internalise a belief that others will judge your mistakes. We must remember that no-one is perfect and that we are all here to live life, whilst being honest with ourselves.

If you prefer to deal with problems on your own, it can be hard to admit to being vulnerable, because you regard it as a sign of weakness.

So we look for confirmation of who we are from other people, such as our family, friends, lovers or companions. They help us build an identity. If you have nobody to mirror back to you, you can feel totally isolated. Yet equally, what is mirrored back is not necessarily who you are: it may just be the habitual responses you have accumulated as a result of the strategies you have devised for getting through life. Your personality is not the essential core of you. Your core is your inner wisdom. When you are in tune with your inner self, it radiates out like a beacon of shining light, just as a baby is a radiant being, taking everything in and giving everything out in an open and receptive way. A baby's sense of identity is not in his or her appearance, but in his or her responses to all the new experiences life is giving them.

The following are some of the remedies I use a lot in my clinics to help people to tune into their core, so that loneliness becomes less of a problem and more joy comes into their life.

AURUM: For people with an intense and idealistic character who feel devastated by the loss of a family member or broken relationship. They criticise themselves a lot and so don't accept themselves as they are. A lot of guilt stored in the back area, hence there are pains there. Energy may be worse at

10 am, with stomach and arthritic type pains.

NAT MUR: Ill effects from anger, a loss or disappointment in their life. They prefer to cry on their own, and find it hard to express their feelings to close family and friends.

PULSATILLA: They feel very sorry for themselves, as if they are the victim, and are unloved and abandoned. They comfort eat a lot to ease their unhappiness. Energy worse from 3 - 5 pm and from 3 - 5 am. PMT (may feel very low before a period, or suffer from breast tenderness).

STRAMONIUM: For people who are fearful as a result of feeling totally alone.

Learn that you are never alone because on a spirit level you are always connected to others. You need to find strength and support within your own being, and to develop a feeling of connectedness. Knowing that we are all going through the same struggle can help you to feel your humanity and to realise that you are not alone.

THE CURE FOR FEAR – PART 1

A contagious disease is spreading like the plague across Ireland at present. I'm sure you've heard of it: it's called "Fear." Fear of not having enough money, fear of losing a job, fear of change, fear of the future and so on.

I remember watching a program with journalist David McWilliams about a year ago where he spoke very negatively about the economy, and said that a recession was coming our way. "The Celtic Tiger is dying a slow death," he said. Many people listened to what he said, and many people spread the negative news. The seeds of a recession had already been sown. This fear of recession created negative thoughts in people's minds. Fear is a limitation of our minds, and all too often what we think is what we get. As an example, I have two clients who are plumbers. Mr Plumber A dwelt on his fear that there might not be enough work for him and his employees, whereas Mr Plumber B stayed fully present, only thinking positive thoughts. Mr A's company has since folded, whereas Mr B's business continues to thrive. Mr A trusted – and continues to trust – that everything is OK.

Nothing comes from outside of us. We are at the centre of everything that happens in our lives. Everything is inside us, every experience, every relationship, every act is the mirror of a mental pattern that we have inside of us. So if you have a fear of change, you always stay put rather than venturing into the unknown – but it may be that the unknown is the very thing you are searching for, and you miss out on the abundance, joy and inner power that a change could bring because you choose to stay stuck.

The base of anger is often fear. For example, when I am preparing for my workshops, I sometimes get angry if things aren't flowing, or if my kids disturb me and get in my way. But my anger is coming from a place of fear – a fear that the workshop won't go as well as I want it to. So anger is a fear that becomes a defence mechanism – we are afraid that something bad might happen. The answer is to acknowledge the emotion associated with the fear, which then breaks its power over us. By working though the fear, you turn the negative emotion into something positive.

Fear can also be a negative emotion that creates a negative experience both inside and outside the body. Love and trust are the opposite of fear. The more we are willing to love and trust who we are, the more we attract an abundance of not just money but also the things that make us feel happy and fulfilled in our daily lives: loving relationships, a rewarding job, positive people around us and so on.

As a wise Buddhist said, "If we capture the small moments, the big moment is always at hand."

In part 2 of this article, I write about more positive ways to dissolve the catching disease called "fear."

THE CURE FOR FEAR – PART 2

In part 1of this article, I wrote of the new contagious disease called fear, and how fear of not having enough money was leading to a ripple effect across the country, affecting companies and self-employed people. As I explained, fear is often a lack of trust in ourselves – and because of that, we do not trust in the flow of life. When we trust, we are letting go of the situation. Many people are afraid of letting go due to a fear of what might happen. But when we do trust and let go, we are tuning into a higher vibration of energy that is so powerful that at this level miracles can happen.

If we do not trust that we are not being taken care of at a higher level, then we feel we must control everything from the physical level. We then automatically feel fear because we cannot control everything in our lives. Trust is what we learn when we want to overcome our fears. It's called taking "the leap of faith."

If the fear gets inside your body – if you ***let*** the fear get inside your body - and it stays lodged there, adrenalin may pump through your body to protect you from danger, leading to palpitations, trembling, panic attacks, insomnia and so on. So learn to observe your fears. Learn to observe your body. And learn to recognise that you are not your fears. Love yourself so that you can take care of yourself. Do everything to strengthen your body and your mind. Do not mask your fears with addictions. Practice deep breathing exercises and affirm daily:

"I am at one with the power that created me. I am safe. All is well in my world."

"I am willing to surrender all my fears and worries to my Creator right now, and when I do so, everything turns out perfectly."

I see many people who fear the future: they are afraid of moving forward, afraid of change, or afraid of impending problems. If only they could trust that change could bring them the very things they want in their lives! But to lose their fear, they first have to change from within. When you dissolve the disease called fear, you accept that no-one is perfect, you acknowledge where you are right now, doing your best, and operating out of love and trust.

I believe that one of the reasons for the current recession is to make people stop looking outwards for answers. Now is a time for reflection, for everyone to look inwardly and ask questions like "Do I need to change myself? Do I need to change my career? Do I need to change my work / life balance?" We forget that the power lies in each and every one of us to change ourselves. When you seek love, happiness and trust, you must work on yourself first, before you can feel comfortable with sharing these things unconditionally with others.

Our thoughts create our reality. Ask yourself: are your thoughts controlling and fear-based, or are they allowing and love-based? It is only by trusting that the contagious disease of fear can be addressed and worked through.

THE POWER OF SELF-EMPOWERMENT

Q: *I am very stressed out. I am a mother with 2 young children and I also have a full time job. I work in a company where I feel I am always burdened with extra work whilst others get off scot-free – I find it difficult to say no. As a result I suffer constant fatigue and headaches. Any advice to help me get out of this rut would be of great help! Thank you.*

A: You have the power within you to do something about your situation. In fact, everyone has this power within them, but not everyone connects to it. If you choose to stay as you are, you will remain stuck. You need to make a conscious decision to stop being the victim, and stop playing the blame game. That is the first step in reclaiming your power.

When you are asked to take on extra work, learn to say "I'm busy at the moment, can you come back later", or simply learn to speak the truth powerfully and lovingly. Say what you really think. Say what you want to say rather than what you think the other person would like to hear. If you are not true to yourself, this can affect your lymphatic system and blood circulation, hence allowing disease to get in, as a result of pent-up emotions of resentment. You will not get respect or appreciation from other people if you don't give it to yourself in the first place. Self empowerment comes from loving yourself. So stop pleasing outwardly and start pleasing yourself more. Have you thought about working part-time? Is it an option? Ask! Also, your boss may think that you are coping very well, but you need to communicate assertively and firmly that delegation of responsibility may be required.

There is more. As a parent, when you empower yourself, your self-worth is automatically mirrored on to your children. If you are empowered, your children will also be empowered with confidence and self-esteem.

When you approach your true needs with courage and power instead of fear, you ignite in yourself a sense of trust. When you speak the truth powerfully and lovingly, your energy flows better in your body and fatigue diminishes. Good luck!

THE POWER OF THE NOW

Q: *I daydream a lot, and often forget where I put things, or why I have gone into a certain room. My memory is not that great, so I was wondering if you have suggestions that might help me.*

A:We all tend to daydream from time to time. We each typically have 60,000 thoughts daily, and it is only when we create space in between these thoughts that we improve our concentration and become more focussed. If you put your keys down and your thoughts are elsewhere, you automatically may not remember where you left them!

An easy first step to connect to the now is to wriggle your toes and acknowledge that you are grounded. I like to imagine that my feet are like the roots of a tree connecting to the earth. This simple technique helps the energy to flow from your head area to your feet, and thus lessens the number of your thoughts and connects you more to the present. Otherwise the racing mind is like a hamster on a wheel, constantly going round and round with one thought chasing the next. These constant – and often unwanted - thoughts can in turn make you feel impatient or frustrated with yourself. Everything needs to be done now, not tomorrow.

Stop worrying about the past or the future. Acknowledge your thoughts but just let them go. The secret to true happiness is living in the present. Try this simple exercise for five minutes every morning:

- **Breathe in deeply and slowly to the count of 1- 2 - 3 (your tummy muscles should rise)**
- **Hold for 1 – 2 – 3**
- **Breathe out slowly to the count of 1- 2 – 3.**

When you bring your mind into your breathing techniques, you immediately reduce the number of thoughts. Your mental clarity and awareness are enhanced. This process also eases emotional tensions, anxieties, irritations and depression. When we relax, our resistance to disease increases. The art of quietening the mind is a tool that we can all use to find the stillness within where there is no suffering, only inner peace.

You could also try the remedy Nux Vomica 30 to detox both the mind and body. Take morning and evening for two weeks, and then let your body do its own healing for two weeks. Nux Vomica helps you to be more patient with both yourself and those around you. I take this remedy if I cannot switch off my thoughts when I am meditating. I find that it helps me to be more patient and more focussed, and it also enhances my concentration and memory.

Try reading the book "The Power of the Now" by Eckhart Tolle. It explains in more depth how to detach yourself from your thoughts and become more empowered as a result.

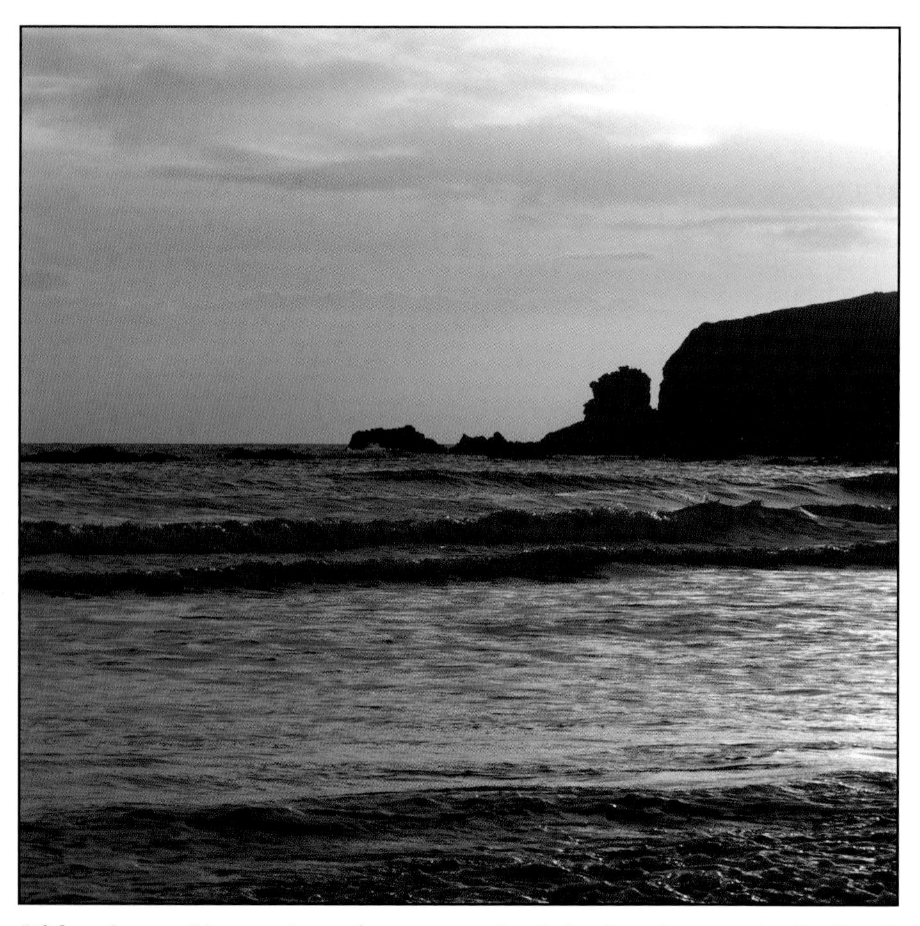

"If there is something you have always wanted to do but have been putting it off until the right time – do it and do it now!"

POSITIVE THINKING & AFFIRMATIONS: INTRO & KEEPING SAFE

I am a great believer in the power of positive thinking – in fact it is something I am passionate about! We all have infinite potential. Within each of us lies the possibility for success, health, beauty and inner peace. However, when we constantly think negative thoughts, we limit or block our potential. But the process can be reversed NOW!

If we choose to focus on failure, we fail. If we hold success in our thoughts, we must inevitably succeed. If we focus on ill health or poverty, we can create such ill health and poverty in our lives that we are crippled by them. If we hold visions of success and wealth, or of health, happiness and love, then these qualities come into our lives.

Most of us want to be joyful, strong, confident, rich and popular, but we don't know how to change the negative beliefs which constantly play in our minds. One of the most effective ways - which I have used successfully for both myself and my clients – is to replace the old beliefs with positive, wholesome ones, and to make daily affirmations. An affirmation is a positive statement about ourselves or our abilities. Once impressed in our unconscious mind, the positive belief manifests in our lives. Affirmations must be done daily, as they must pass through the critical censor before they reaches the unconscious mind.

The unconscious mind is where we hold our belief system, so it is only when affirmations become fixed in the unconscious that we can change our beliefs and therefore our thoughts and our lives. Remember, our thoughts are our health and our riches. An excellent book on this topic is "A Little Light on Spiritual Laws" by Diana Cooper. Here are some wonderfully therapeutic affirmations she uses for keeping safe:

- **"Protected by my inner glow, I am safe wherever I go"**
- **"I grow stronger and stronger every day, Safe and secure in every way"**
- **"I'm guarded and guided, My needs all provided"**
- **"My inner light strong and steady, I am safe and I am ready"**

- **"I'm safe and secure, Guided and sure"**
- **"I feel very strong, For I know I belong"**

I used positive affirmations when I was in my 20's to help me override feelings of depression and constant fatigue in both mind and body. I still use them 20 years on, and have never needed to take anti-depressants since. Used on a daily basis morning and evening, affirmations can change our thought patterns and make them more positive.

When I find that certain clients are very stuck in their negative thought patterns, I get them to write down their individual affirmations in accordance with where their own energies are blocked. As an example, one lady I saw had very low physical and mental energy. She kept getting chest infections which antibiotics were not shifting. Using iridology, I saw she had a ring of harmony in her eyes, which indicated that she wanted peace at all times even to the detriment of her body. She resented life and hence ate "poor me" foods like chocolate and cheese which only served to bring her energy levels down even further. So together we drew up a personalised list of positive affirmations, as follows:

"I love myself more."
"It is OK for me to say no to people."
"I listen to my body's needs, and allow myself to rest when I need to."

Within two weeks, she called me to say that her energy levels had risen, and that she felt much more relaxed in herself. In time, her chest infections also cleared up, and she became a much happier person – living proof of the power of positive affirmations!

POSITIVE THINKING & AFFIRMATIONS: HAPPINESS

Affirmations must always be in the present tense. Life is a series of here and now moments. Our unconscious mind, which is like a computer, has no concept of time, so for it, tomorrow never comes.

Affirmations must only contain positive words. If we affirm that we are letting go of greed, our computer focuses on greed. So instead we must concentrate on the positivity of generosity. Likewise, if we focus on anger, we are concentrating on something negative. Instead, choose to focus on love: this will help to dissolve all anger in your cells, and thus to reduce disease in your body.

Affirmations do not use the word "not". The unconscious mind cannot take in negatives. Check it out. Close your eyes and say "I don't want to see a chocolate bar." The only picture your unconscious mind can present to you is a yummy chocolate bar! So if you affirm that you don't want a cigarette, you are presenting your mind with a picture of one, and will crave a smoke. Instead, affirm the positive benefits of health and the joy of eating wholesome, fresh fruit.

My all time favourite affirmation for happiness is as follows:

"I tune into my joy, happiness, laughter and love, and share them outwardly."

Repeat it to yourself three times every morning and evening for two weeks. If you can say it out loud, all the better. Be very clear in what you want and affirm it in the present tense. Say it daily, be patient, and it will present itself to you when the time is right.

As proof of the power of positive affirmations, here's an example from my own life. I had been in my Kilkenny clinic in a small cottage for four years and knew it was time to move on to bigger premises. My landlady was very patient and kind. She needed to do major repairs to the cottage's roof but she could not do so whilst I was holding my clinics there. At the time I was very busy with my clinics and my family life, and did not have the time to seek out and view potential new premises. So I decided to put the affirmations to the test. I affirmed "I now work in a spacious, light-filled, affordable clinic in town."

Within months, the clinic came to me, and better still it was only 4 doors down from my existing premises. So it was an easy move to a more spacious, light-filled, newly decorated and affordable clinic!

RECONNECTING TO JOY & HAPPINESS

Are lightness, laughter and fun all missing in your life? Are you taking your life too seriously? Just take a look around you – work is serious, life is serious, sports, the news, education, relationships, parenting ... all so serious. Even food and sexuality, two joyous gifts that are meant to be fun, have become serious stuff.

So is it any wonder that people feel so guilty about indulging in a piece of chocolate, because even the simple pleasure of eating it has been taken away. We seem to have lost our ability to enjoy the simplest things in life. And it gets worse. Ask yourself – does other people's laughter - or other people's enjoyment - bother you? If the answer is yes, then you are truly disconnected from your own joy.

Most of us simply don't spend enough time appreciating what we have achieved or what we have in our lives. Instead, we focus on what we haven't done or what needs to be done. By our own choice, we choose struggle instead of joy. But true success in life comes from noticing and appreciating all the blessings around us. So what can be done to reconnect to the joy in our lives?

Put simply, we need to allow our natural flow of energy to emerge. In our modern-day, non-stop lives, we compensate by going for thrills in any way we can ... which goes some way in explaining our addictions to alcohol, cigarettes, food, drugs and crime. All these things are ultimately self-destructive and are in direct opposition to the connection to the joy and happiness which is rightly ours to own. Joy and happiness do not need to be money-oriented. You can reconnect to your joy through a simple pleasure, like a walk in nature, dancing to your favourite song, playing a musical instrument, singing, or weeding a patch in your garden. By doing so, you step off the merry go round for once, relax your busy mind, and draw in the universal energy that surrounds you.

So what steps can you take to connect to joy in your life? Here are some simple suggestions:

LOVE YOURSELF!

When you learn to accept yourself as you are, it becomes easier to love yourself. Start by loving yourself first, then extend this towards your family and friends, and bring love into all aspects of your life. Such positive thought patterns will also boost the energy levels in your body and help it to heal itself.

STOP WORRYING!
When you worry, you invite fearful things to happen in your life: this is the universal law of attraction. When you worry about someone, you are the instigator of negativity towards them and their situation. Instead of worrying, just say "I let go of the situation, I trust and send love and light towards it." This positive thought pattern allows the situation to be dissolved, even though you felt like it was out of your control.

DO WHAT MAKES YOU HAPPY!
If you know what makes you feel happy, ask yourself – "why am I denying myself the chance of joy?" The only person stopping you is you! Tune into your creativity and your inner voice - and start enjoying yourself.

STOP LIVING TOO MUCH IN THE HEAD!
Sometimes people are too caught up in their minds or in the hectic pace of day to day living. Take time in your life to slow down and focus on simply "being" for once. Meditate. Sit on a park bench and watch the world go by. Look at the wonderful world of nature around you. Get out of your head, get into your body and enjoy the small moments in life.

FOCUS ON THE GOOD THINGS IN YOUR LIFE!
Instead of worrying about what you don't have or what you haven't done, write a "Gratitude Journal" of all the positive things you have in your life. The next time you are feeling down, take out your journal to remind yourself that life is not so bad!

BREAK THE OLD THOUGHT PATTERNS & EMPOWER YOURSELF!
Some people resist change and choose to stay stuck in their own habits, resisting change. So stop choosing to be the victim, stop feeling sorry for yourself, and stop choosing to connect to the pain in your life. By empowering yourself and refusing to give sway to your negative thought patterns, you break the power and the hold they have over you.

GET TO KNOW YOURSELF BETTER!
One of my clients told me that she loved to play golf. However, she was so competitive that the need to win had completely overtaken her joy in playing.

I advised her to take an objective look at herself: she could not see that her over-competitiveness was ruining her enjoyment of the game. On her next visit, she told me that for the first time whilst playing golf, she had heard the birds singing, and had taken in the sheer joy of nature all around her on the course. She was exhilarated and cured of her anxiety, but still played her best game.

These are all very simple examples, but they are no less valid for being so! So take a few minutes to get away from your busy schedule and write yourself a list of what you are going to do to reconnect to your joy – and then just do it!

STEPS TO CREATE JOY & PEACE OF MIND

Elsewhere I have written about the possible links between high cholesterol / heart problems and a lack of love and joy in our lives. So here's a series of positive steps you can take to bring more happiness and joy in your life (and who knows – maybe reduce your cholesterol levels too!):

- **Forgive yourself.**
- **Be honest and true with yourself.**
- **Speak the truth powerfully and lovingly when required. Speak with integrity at all times.**
- **Love yourself more and live according to your inner guidance.**
- **Be kind to yourself and kind to others.**
- **Practice meditation, yoga and positive affirmations regularly.**
- **Eat simple, healthy foods, and avoid toxins like alcohol, cigarettes, sugar, tea, coffee and so on.**
- **Maintain healthy sleep habits and patterns.**
- **Avoid negative people and negative media.**
- **Let go of your problems and surrender them to God.**
- **Walk in nature regularly.**
- **Simplify your life.**
- **Say "No" when you need to – in other words, empower yourself.**
- **Don't take things too personally.**
- **Stop making assumptions.**
- **Do your best at all times, even when you fail.**
- **Be mindful of conflicts.**
- **Choose to heal yourself by empowering yourself.**
- **Live more in the now and enjoy the present moment.**
- **Bring humour and laughter into your life.**
- **Take responsibility for where you are at. You may not be the cause of the problem, but you are the only one who can resolve it.**

- **Always work on solutions to your problems: this brings in positive energy. Remember: problems are negative energy.**

9
POT LUCK!

A DOG'S LIFE

When my father died some years ago, I bought my mother a Yorkshire Terrier to keep her company. I bought the terrier in Tralee, and thus just had to call her Rosie, after the Rose of Tralee! A few years later, just before I got married, Rosie had a charming puppy called Sammy. We never did find out who the father was, but from the look of Sammy, it must have been a collie from one of the neighbouring farms. As soon as I saw Sammy on our family farm in County Galway, I knew there was no way I was going back to my job in London without him. So the next month when I got married, Sammy Dog was part of the package. It was just as well my husband loves dogs too! – indeed he used to joke that he knew how long we'd been married by working out Sammy's age! With our family pet Sammy Dog, we shared the pleasure of almost 15 years of wonderful companionship, loyalty, walks, holidays, laughter and joy. We have four kids, but we always considered Sammy as our first born, and he was like a big brother to our children (which, of course, he was). He also kept us in touch with nature when we took him for his walks twice a day.

To our great sorrow and sadness, Sammy passed away a few days before Christmas. As we struggled to come to terms with his death, we tried to focus on the happy memories of our times together. And it struck me that dogs can teach us so many life lessons. A dog gives us unconditional love at all times, even if they are abused or neglected. A dog is always there to welcome you with a wag of the tail or to cheer you up when you are feeling down. Dog owners have a common bond - I have made many friends from talking to fellow dog walkers. And it broke our hearts when one of our daughters said "I'd give all of my presents back if we could get Sammy back for Christmas" – her words really put the over-commercialism of Christmas into perspective.

I once saw a lady in my clinic who was very lonely and nervous about living on her own. She lived inside her house and her dog lived outside. Having grown up on a farm in Galway, I know that we Irish often keep our dogs outside, but I advised her to uncondition her programming and to bring her dog inside for the winter months. This she did, and when I saw her some time later, she said that having her dog indoors made her feel more secure, more relaxed and less lonely. Indeed, there is medical evidence to suggest that stroking a pet reduces people's blood pressure and makes them feel calmer in themselves.

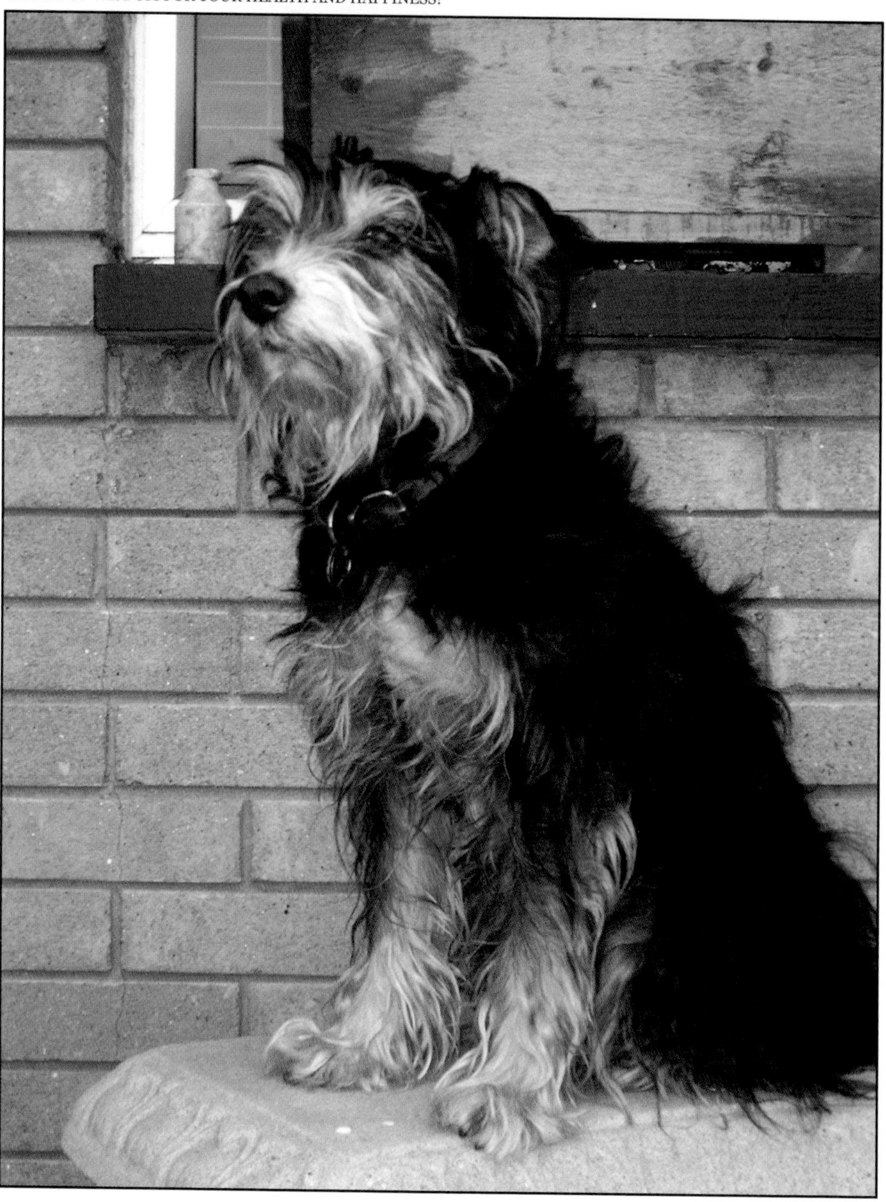

Sammy

We have so many happy memories of Sammy: playing Frisbee, bounding into view as we walked through fields where the grass was three times his height, running into the waves and then away from them as they came in, barking joyously when he found a ball or something interesting, watching his hair-raising hairstyles when he was wet or when it was windy, seeing him trying to eat snowballs, chasing (but never quite catching) the cats who dared to invade his garden ... He lived with us for ten years in London, before coming back to Ireland five years ago, and in all that time he was truly part of the family.

Sammy's passing has taught me and my family that sadness and grief can be used positively to acknowledge your loss, to recognise your sensitivity, and to accept that it is OK to cry - as the old saying goes, "For every tear shed, a day is added to your life." We all experience pain and loss in our lives from the passing of a loved one, be it a person or a pet. But I strongly believe that for every pain, it can be turned around, acknowledged and worked through. Our son wrote a beautiful poem the day after Sammy's passing, full of happy memories. I have always believed that if you can, being able to celebrate and smile at the good times - and not becoming bogged down in the sadness associated with a loss - is immensely beneficial, and helps us to come to terms with a bereavement. Nowadays, most people live too much in their heads, rushing everywhere, never stopping, and with little or no time for anything or anyone. When we experience things like grief or sadness, it makes us slow down, reflect, and connect with our hearts. When we start listening to our hearts, we empathise more with other people, we become more compassionate, and we judge less.

I met a kind man when walking Sammy in Thomastown a few weeks before he died, and this man said to me "You know, I feel there is more to dogs than meets the eye." And you know, I agree with him. A dog doesn't ask for much, but if you show him respect and appreciation, he will repay you with unconditional love and loyalty. So please remember, if you were lucky enough to get a dog or puppy for Christmas, that it is your responsibility to feed it, walk it and love it ... do this and you will see the rewards come back to you tenfold.

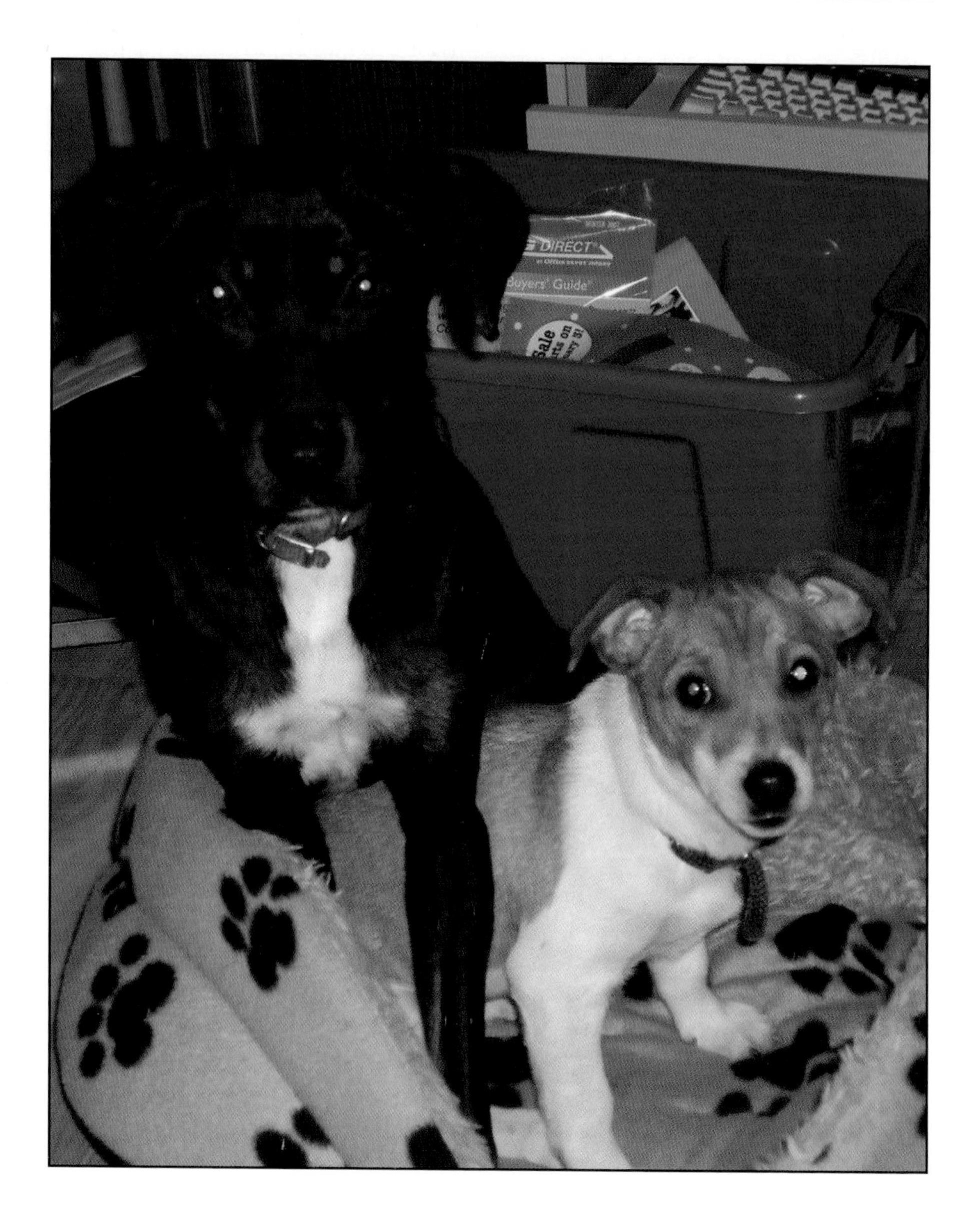

Sunny & Oscar

A POEM FOR OSCAR

Regular readers of my newspaper columns will know that I am great lover of animals. The previous article is about our much-loved dog Sammy, who died aged 15 just before Christmas. In January, although we were still missing Sammy terribly, we took on two new dogs from the Inistioge Puppy Rescue Centre: Sunny, a boisterous and bouncy cross of we know not what parentage, and Oscar, an initially shy but then wonderfully welcoming and smiling Jack Russell. Sunny and Oscar were great fun, and helped to heal our memories of Sammy.

Sadly, five months after he came into our lives, Oscar was run over. Our only consolation was that he was killed instantly and did not suffer. My husband wrote a beautiful poem about Oscar for our children, and I am sharing it here, in the hope that it might be of comfort to anyone who has lost a much loved pet recently:

Even the skies cried a million tears, the day you were taken away
But the clouds gave way to a beautiful sunset to speed you on your way
Here one moment and gone the next, you left us far too soon
And we'd give anything to bring you back – the sun, the stars, the moon.

We'll always remember you with a smile, the way you used to run
When you came to us - so serious, when you left us - so much fun
Running, laughing, jumping, barking, with your best friend Sunny
And in the small basket by the computer desk, you were really more than funny.

We know that you're in heaven now, but your spirit's with us still
We know you're watching over us, and know you always will
We know that time will heal the pain, and tears will turn to laughter
And you'll stay in that special place in our hearts for ever, ever after.

Though you were only here for a short time, you left us memories for a lifetime
Only here for a short while, but you left us with a big smile
And though we're sad you left us, we're so glad that you came
Our thoughts of you will shine for all time, like an everlasting flame.

To end this story on a happier note, we now have a new friend for Sunny – Sylvie, a collie spaniel cross.

EMBRACE LIFE AND ACCEPT DEATH

The journey of life begins with birth and ends with death. You may fear death because it takes away everything - everything that you love and everything that you own. But rich or poor, from the highest to the lowest, death is inevitable for us all. When you know someone who dies, someone close to you, whom you loved and cared for, their passing will naturally cause you great pain, sadness and suffering. Grieving is a rite of passage and a process we must all go through at some stage in our lives. But for some people, the pain continues without end, and there is no release. Every anniversary, every birthday, every Christmas brings up more pain. When this happens, you may resist moving on and connecting to your own inner joy.

In his song Voyage, Christy Moore sang: "Life is an ocean and love is a boat - In troubled waters, it keeps us afloat." And yes, love can keep us afloat. We are all part of the big ocean, on the same journey. Sometimes we separate from the ocean, but we are all part of the bigger picture called "Life and Death" and we always ultimately return to the ocean and the boat. The boat can represent many things – love for yourself, the love of your close family and friends who are always there to support you through a painful time, or simply the act of being kinder to yourself during a time of loss.

In times of sorrow, sadness and loss, real friendship always shows its true colours. Even if it's just a handshake, a hug or a "How are you?" it shows that people really do care and can connect to each other. But whilst the comfort of friends and family can and does help us to work through the grieving process, I believe we also need to consider the two cords of life to truly reconnect to our inner joy.

The first cord is the cord of love that never dies. It will always be connected to your loved ones, you never lose it, it always stays with you, and it helps to heal the pain of separation. I'm sure if a departed loved one could come back, they would say, "Please don't feel guilty about what-ifs and what-might-have-been's – just rejoice in the good times we had together and get on with living your life positively."

The second cord is the psychic cord. This is the cord that holds you back from getting on with your own life. This is the cord of guilt, of pain and of rejection. If you have been suffering from a bereavement for too long, this is the cord you need to cut. In your mind, picture as big a pair of scissors as you can, then cut the psychic cord and let it go. The cord of love will help you in this process. The cord of love never dies, it helps your heart to remove the armour that surrounds it, to lift your energy, and to make you feel more alive and connected to yourself. Remember: the chord of love empowers you.

To close, here are two beautiful quotations, the first by the Lebanese American poet Kahlil Gibran, and the second by an unknown author:

"When you are sorrowful, look again in your heart, and you shall see that in truth you are weeping for that which has been your delight."

"Love is stronger than death even though it can't stop death from happening, but no matter how hard death tries it can't separate people from love. It can't take away our memories either. In the end, life is stronger than death."

FRENCH LESSONS!

My husband Jerry looks after our four kids full time and also the business side of my clinics. Every so often he takes a break on his own to recharge the batteries. He recently went to Biarritz, lucky him, and he came back enthusing about the place and his few days away in this south-western coastal corner of France. We discussed over dinner why he had had such a good time, and I thought I would share his thoughts, as they have some good advice and tips for all of us:

All the shops still close for lunch! Good for them – this used to be the case in Ireland, but creeping commercialism has put paid to our valiant workers always getting a break. If France can survive with lunch breaks and closed shops, why can't we? (and on a similar note, whatever happened to early day closing?!). I'm delighted to say that where I live in Thomastown, people still take their lunch breaks, and no matter how busy I am, I always take mine!

No mobile for four days: he had his mobile with him, but he switched it off and didn't go anywhere near it. He said the sense of freedom and relief was palpable! Whenever I go for a walk in nature, I always leave my mobile at home – this helps me to be more fully present with the beauty and sounds of nature. So why not try and be mobile free for one day a week?

The place is beautifully clean and litter free: it's often only when you go away from Ireland that you realise what a problem we have with litter. We have a truly beautiful country, so why can't we Irish learn to take more care of our most precious natural resource? I was in Tramore recently, and was shocked by the amount of rubbish there – it made me ashamed to be Irish. It's not the council's fault – people should take responsibility for their own rubbish!

The locals are wonderfully welcoming and friendly: we are lucky in the South-East that we still have many friendly people in our shops and in general – but it is noticeable that we are not as friendly as we used to be. Don't forget your smiles and your good mornings – they are an integral part of life!

The old couples stroll hand in hand along the promenade in the evenings: what a lovely thought! Love never dies, so next time you are out with your husband or wife, young or old, why don't you demonstrate your love and hold hands!

Sea air is great for your health: I couldn't agree more – there is something wonderfully refreshing, invigorating and yet relaxing about sea air that seems to make us feel more positive and happier, and leads to a good night's sleep. If it's been a while since you went to the coast, why not dust off those flip flops and take a trip to see the sea, especially now the good weather is coming back.

Doing nothing is great! He spent a large part of his break just sitting on the sea-front watching the waves and the world go by. We spend so much of our lives rushing around, always doing something, that we forget how refreshing and revitalising it is to simply sit and do nothing – when was the last time you did it?

The next time we get one of our rare and precious weekends away together without the kids, we are going to try and go to Biarritz. So if you see a middle-aged couple there strolling along the prom hand in hand, it might just be us!

LET THE SUN SHINE FROM WITHIN!

It seems the big topic of discussion at the moment – other than the recession – is that old Irish staple – the weather! "What terrible weather we're having! – not more rain! – isn't it cold for summer!" – and so on. Some people say the bad summer weather gets them down. Last week I heard someone say "I would be happier if the sun was shining" – and it's true – a spell of good weather does indeed seem to make everyone happier.

All of this made me think of when my family and I were in Clonea last summer with our caravan. It rained ceaselessly for three days, and we had forgotten to pack our wellies. The kids had such fun and laughter running and jumping in the mud, and then they would run down to the beach and practice their surfing. In spite of the rain, it was one of the happiest memories of the summer holidays.

We own two dogs, and regardless of the weather, they have to be walked twice daily. Yesterday, whilst walking in the local meadow, I counted nearly two dozen butterflies. It was such a pretty sight to see them all in various colours, hues and sizes. This sight brought me such joy and happiness that I felt as if the sun was shining inside of me. It brought a smile to my face, as walks in nature always do. In spite of the bad weather we've been having, the swallows still fly, the butterflies still flutter, and the flowers still grow.

Inside each and every individual, there is an energy that shines just as brightly as the sun that shines in the sky. This energy is called joy and happiness. All we have to do is to tap into it daily by doing something – no matter how small – that makes us happy. For me, this means my daily runs and walks in nature. Doing what makes me happy makes my sun shine from within.

So don't let the bad weather get you down. Just practice daily being connected to your own inner sun, and when the sun in the sky isn't shining, you will still feel bright and happy. What's more, you will find your inner sunshine will also reflect brightly into the lives of those around you. To close, here's a few lines by the American poet Henry Wadsworth Longfellow:

"Kind hearts are the gardens, kind thoughts are the roots,
Kind words are the flowers, kind deeds are the fruits,
Take care of your garden, and keep out the weeds,
Fill it with sunshine, kind words and kind deeds."

THE DRAINERS!

Q: *I have a friend who never stops complaining. If it's not her health, it's her family, or her workmates, or the weather etc. Now I know we all have our bad days – but hers seem to be every day! How as a friend can I help her? We used to be really good pals, but now I find myself not wanting to see her, plus I always seem to have a headache after visiting her! Please help me save our friendship!*

A: You'd be surprised how often people ask me the best way to deal with people like your friend – or the "drainers" as I call them. You really are a true friend to want to help her, and I admire your unconditional and compassionate nature. But as you yourself said, she is obviously affecting your physical body - hence the headaches. So my advice follows below. Here we are talking about a negative friend, but you can also use some of these tips for other negative people in your life, eg relatives, workmates etc:

- **Make sure that you are in good form yourself before visiting your friend. If you're in bad form, don't visit her, or you will simply end up with a worse headache than usual.**
- **Protect yourself before your visit. Visualise a white light surrounding your body, and feel that nothing can permeate this white light. In other words, her negative energy stays outside your body and doesn't get inside and affect you. This tip really does work!**
- **Try the mirror trick. Visualise a mirror between you and your friend, with the mirror facing her. Everything negative that comes out of her mouth gets reflected back to her, sadly meaning that she will be the one that gets the headache.**
- **Don't feed into her negativity. When she starts to complain, consciously maintain your own energy, and change the topic to something more positive. Don't gossip, as this just accumulates negative energy and you may both end up with a headache.**
- **Given you are so caring about your friendship and so thoughtful towards your friend, why not buy or lend her a positive living book, eg "The Power of Positive Thinking" by Norman Peale. If she is insulted, then maybe she isn't such a good friend after all.**
- **Work on bringing up your own energy by doing things you really enjoy,**

like gardening, dancing, singing, walking in nature etc.

- **If you feel things are becoming too extreme, simply see her less often, or even not at all. Your own health is more important!**

You see, some people simply enjoy being miserable – they feel they can get more sympathy from their family and friends. Perhaps she doesn't want to change. Old habits die hard, and she may wish to remain the victim, happily wallowing in her misery. Maybe in your own space and territory you might feel more empowered to speak your truth powerfully and lovingly to her, and still maintain your friendship. Remember, if your own energy is good, the truth will come out more positively. You might consider using the Positive - Negative - Positive truth statement. Positive: "I really like you as a person and value our close friendship," Negative: "But it's getting me down when we talk about negative things all the time," Positive: "So let's get back to how things used to be, when we used to laugh and joke and be happy when we talked." People usually latch on to the positive first, and are more prepared for the negative truth when it comes. Good luck, isn't she lucky to have a friend like you.

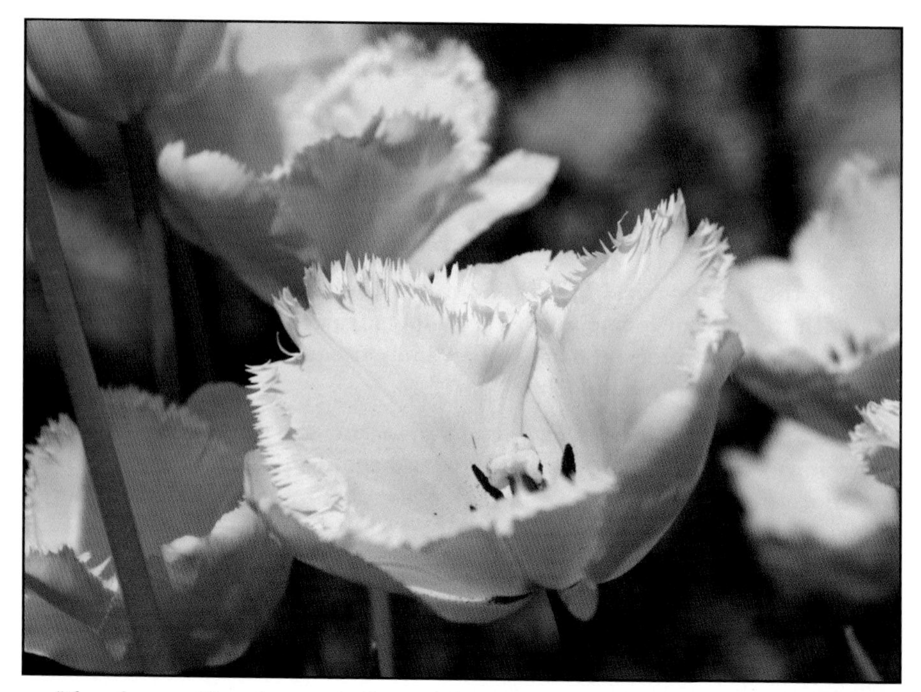

"If you have nothing pleasant at all to say about someone, it is best to say nothing at all."

THE BABY STARLING

Last weekend I was in the playground with my kids when I witnessed a sickening act. Three young teenage boys there appeared to be kicking a stone around – only the stone turned out to be a baby starling. One boy continued to laugh and chase his friends around with bird in hand. I was adamant that it couldn't be a bird, but my kids insisted it was, so we followed the boys until they let the bird drop. Sure enough it was a helpless baby starling, eyes blinking and barely breathing. I could see that its chances of survival were slim, as some of its internal organs were external. But life is life. We took the bird home with us, gave it some drops of water, kept it warm, and even tried to feed it a worm. It survived for two hours.

This sorry incident set me thinking - there were two guilty parties in this story. Obviously the boy who was being cruel to the bird, but also his two friends who stood by and did nothing. Were they too weak to show that they cared? Did peer pressure from the other boy make them feel the need to kick a helpless bird just for a laugh? It may just have been a helpless bird, but how would the boys have felt if they were down-trodden and weak, and somebody felt like kicking them around?

If the main perpetrator possessed a strong sense of love inside of him, he would not have felt the need to use an innocent victim of a baby bird to be more approved of by his friends. And perhaps the two bystanders felt inside as helpless as the poor starling.

As parents, we have a great responsibility to ignite empowerment in our children. Do we conform to outside pressure and go along with the crowd, or do we speak the truth as we know it? Our morals for love and respect start in the home place. As parents we can only guide our children. They learn by example. They witness our love for ourselves, the love between Mum & Dad, love for siblings, and of course, love for all aspects of life. Nobody's the perfect parent. We can only hope to guide our children in the hope that they will grow their own wings with respect for all species of life.

RECOMMENDED FURTHER READING

I am often asked by my clients to recommend books for certain ailments or circumstances. Here is a list of some of my favourite complementary health books and positive living books. I've consciously only chosen one book by each author, but would strongly recommend anything written by Deepak Chopra, Dr Wayne Dyer, Patrick Francis, Louise Hay, Doreen Virtue, Jan de Vries and Gary Zukav.

- Golden Day by Robert Burdette
- The Secret by Rhonda Byrne
- The Complete Homeopathy Handbook by Miranda Castro
- Candida Albicans by Leon Chaitlow
- The Book of Secrets by Deepak Chopra
- A Little Light on Spiritual Laws by Diana Cooper
- Your Erroneous Zones by Dr Wayne Dyer
- The Grand Design I to V by Patrick Francis
- Excuse Me, Is This Your Body? by Abbas Ghadmi
- You Can Heal Your Life by Louise L. Hay
- The Hay Diet by Dr William Hay
- Ask & It Is Given by Esther & Jerry Hicks
- Born to Heal by Tony Hogan
- The Art of Power by Thich Naht Hanh
- The Power of Positive Thinking by Norman Peale
- The Four Agreements by Don Miguel Ruiz
- The Bodymind Workbook by Debbie Shapiro
- The Power of the Now by Eckhart Tolle
- Healing with Angels by Doreen Virtue
- The Nature Doctor by Dr H C Vogel
- Stress & Nervous Disorders by Jan de Vries
- The Seat of the Soul by Gary Zukav

USEFUL ADDRESSES

Irish School of Homeopathy
Dublin
Tel: 01 8682581
www.homoeopathy.ie

Nelson's Homeopathic Pharmacy
15 Duke St
Dublin 2
Tel: 01 6790451
www.nelsonshomeopathy.com

Irish Society of Homeopaths
Galway
Tel: 091 565040
www.irishhomeopathy.ie

Helios Homeopathic Pharmacy (UK)
www.helios.co.uk

Ainsworths Homeopathic Pharmacy (UK)
www.ainsworths.com

Roger Dyson Homeopathy / Diagnostic Kinesiology
www.traditional-health.co.uk
Tel: 00 44 20 8659 5001

John Andrews Iridology
www.johnandrewsiridology.net
Tel: 00 44 1482 222089

Irish Institute of Iridologists
www.iridologyireland.ie

College of Naturopathic Medicine
www.naturopathy.ie
Tel: 01 235 3094

Dr. Patricia O'Toole, GP
23 Staplestown Road,
Carlow
Tel: 059 913 2525

Breda Gardner Homeopathy / Iridology / Diagnostic Kinesiology
Insight Natural Health Clinic
15 Upper Patrick St
Kilkenny
Tel: 056 7724429

Health Therapies Clinic
13 Gladstone St.,
Waterford
Tel: 051 858584

www.bredagardner.com
Email: breda@bredagardner.com